Electrical Nutrition

by
Denie & Shelley Hiestand

ELECTRICAL NUTRITION
By Denie & Shelley Hiestand
ISBN # 0-9684928-1-9

Copyright 1999. All rights reserved.

Printed in Canada.
3rd Update Printing - August 2000

Published in Canada by:
ShellDen Corp.,
101-1001 W Broadway #341
Vancouver BC. V6H 4E4
Canada.

Published in the U.S.A. by:
ShellDen Corp.,
100 Warren Street, Suite 1402
Jersey City, NJ 07302
U.S.A.

Cover Art By Alex Grey.

Design and Printing by Scribe Graphics Inc. (250) 480-4000

Warning - Disclaimer

Electrical Nutrition and Denie Hiestand.

How to stop degeneration and start regeneration so we can live a full and happy life.

Electrical Nutrition is a new way of looking at health based on the electrical construct of the human body and Denie Hiestand's background in engineering, agriculture and knowledge gained from years of clinical experience working with thousands of international clients. He has the ability to explain difficult concepts in an easy, logical way that allows you to work towards perfect health.

Denie has the ability to tune into and become aware of the electrical functions of the body at a deep level, both cellular and electrical, seeing the electrical malfunctions and ascertaining the causes of dis-ease states developing. In Electrical Nutrition and his clinical work, Denie addresses not only the electrical and physical manifestation, but also, the contributing emotional, spiritual, nutritional and lifestyle factors.

Denie Hiestand is an internationally published author, Vibrational Medicine specialist, teacher and healer, with qualifications in six different healing art modalities. He is founder and Dean of the International Academy of Vibrational Medical Science, which has teaching facilities in the United States, Canada, New Zealand and Switzerland.

Denie brings a much sought after experience and knowledge to advanced healing techniques and understanding of the electrical circuitry of the human body. Often referred to as the "Body Electrician" Denie strives to enlighten the medical community and humanity about the importance of the body's electrical circuitry, its repair and maintenance, and the everlasting benefits of honoring your inner self.

Recognized as one of the world's most powerful healers, Denie Hiestand also incorporates in his writing, lectures and courses a very deep understanding of how to live life to the fullest, to follow one's heart, to be in joy and be all you can be.

DEDICATION

To Frank Reglin and Mel and Kathy Tarry, for having the vision and strength to follow your truth. To all the thousands of clients that I have seen over the years that have allowed me to put my theories into practice and enabled me to learn and understand the truth of my own convictions. For this I thank you...
And to Shelley, for your unwavering love and your passion for life that is my inspiration. Thank you my love.

Denie

*I would like to dedicate this new edition to my father, one of the most inspirational heart-centered dedicated men on this planet who died suddenly last year. I wish he had understood earlier the power and wisdom of **Electrical Nutrition**. He was one of the fittest, sportiest, seemingly healthiest people in existence yet he died way before his time with 85% clogged arteries, even though he had been completely replumbed nine years earlier (with six major bypasses of the heart). So, fitness and the recommended Heart Foundation diet didn't work in his case. If only he had listened to Denie, cut out the grains and stopped mixing the crude proteins and carbohydrates together, perhaps he would still be alive today. Instead his diet, which is pretty typical for most westerners, consisted of toast in the morning (bread), a sandwich for lunch (more bread), meat and potatoes for dinner (EEK! bad food combining) and another piece of toast before going to sleep and people wonder why his arteries became blocked!!! May **Electrical Nutrition** be an inspiration to all of humanity, to see beyond the falsehoods and misinformation so prevalent in today's world and realize the truth of these words. Denie has the ability to tell it how it really is with a simplicity and clarity so hard to find. His passion keeps my own fire burning and inspires me to share my light and joy with you all. Thank you Denie for your love and a togetherness people search lifetimes for, that we have rediscovered and are now able to allow to flow in our life's work. I am eternally grateful for this wonderful gift called LIFE.*

Shelley

ACKNOWLEDGEMENTS

A special thank you to John Gray, Ph.D., for your wonderful support of the work that we do. We are eternally grateful and blessed to know you.

Thanks also to Alex Grey for permission to use your artwork on the front cover. It is so energetically tuned-in with our subject matter and has literally been jumping off the shelves at people!

To Dr. Stephen Vizzard, PhD., P.S., Bellevue, Washington; Dr. Kim Kimball, MD, Everett, Washington; Dr. Keith Mumby, PhD., Manchester, England; Peter Baumann, PhD., Switzerland; Dr. Linda C. Hole, MD, Spokane, Washington, Dr. Paula Baruffi, ND, Bellevue, Washington; Dr. Alex Mazurin, ND, Penticton, British Columbia; and to Dr. David Elliot for his book "Electrical Universe," for when I read this book I yelled out with glee, "There is somebody else who understands!" Also, thank you to all the other medical people with whom I have worked over the last 15 years and who have had the patience to stand my unceasing questions, to be a willing and sometimes not so willing partner in passionate debates about how the body works. I would especially like to thank Judy Kubrak, for her incredible medical research information and to Robert Kalan, who generously contributed his editing skills. Also, to the thousands of nameless authors, nameless only because of my inability to remember your names, whose insights have allowed me to piece together my own reality. Without all the work that has preceded me and all the knowledge that is already in existence, I would not be able to share my knowing. Finally, to Shelley, whose fingers titillated our laptop, typing and correcting my flow of words. Her in-depth questioning sometimes drove me nuts, but forced me to analyze my truth and pushed me to explain the logic of my knowing. Thank you Shelley. This book would have been years longer in the making without you.

TABLE OF CONTENTS

MYTHS AND MEDICAL MISCONCEPTIONS

Vibrant health is our birthright - This is not a particle universe - This is an electrical universe - There is no separation - Modern medicine is not "traditional" - Prescription drugs electrically bombard the body - Drugs are toxins - The ancient tradition of massage - The Chinese understanding - Herbs - Take back your power!

NOURISHMENT - AN ELECTRICAL PROCESS

Food either nourishes us or poisons us - Digestion is an electrical process - Correct fermentation is necessary for full life force - Don't mix the proteins (meat) with carbohydrates (bread) and why - How food nourishes us - Disease is an electrical malfunction - Free radical scavengers - Heart disease and Alzheimers - The effect of preservatives and chemically laced foods - Sugar, an electrical time bomb.

THE ROCK TO ROT THEORY

The vibratory rate of foods - The higher the vibration, the more available and alive it is - Rock is the slowest vibration - Animal flesh is the highest vibration - We need electrically alive protein.

VEGETARIANS' ELECTRICAL NONSENSE

Killing with honor - Vegetables are alive too - Everything contains a consciousness - Carrots scream louder than cows - Prime beef is good - Spirulina, a protein source, but it is alive - Tofu, an electrical disaster.

Foreword by John Gray, Ph.D.

Many people search for fulfillment and happiness in their lives, alone and with a partner. Denie and Shelley are two people who live and breathe vitality and aliveness. *Electrical Nutrition* offers practical, insightful information about how we can all gain more health and vitality.

I have personally been interested in health and healing for many years, and it has been refreshing to meet Denie and Shelley and become familiar with their work. They take an unapologetic stance and have the courage to state many things that challenge commonly accepted beliefs. Blatant though it can be, Denie explains a truth from an energy perspective that very few people perceive. He takes what could be called *medical intuitiveness* straight into the realms of full conscious reality. He walks a fine line somewhere between being overly provocative and genuinely concerned about the future of humanity's health.

Electrical Nutrition will certainly wake people up and get them thinking about what is real and what is true for them. Denie's down-to-earth logic is undeniable. He explains his seemingly outrageous concepts in a very realistic, accessible way so that no confusion remains. He offers a lot of practical suggestions of what people can do on a daily basis to increase their energy levels and get more out of life. Once you are happy with your own health, then it is a lot easier to attract what you want into your life.

Denie and Shelley embody *Electrical Nutrition*. They are full of health and vitality and make the most of every opportunity, enjoying every experience. It is a blessing to know them both. I highly recommend *Electrical Nutrition* to anyone interested in pursuing vibrant health and happiness. It may rock your foundations, but sometimes that's a good thing. Read it and see for yourself.

John Gray, Ph.D., Author
Men Are from Mars, Women Are from Venus

INTRODUCTION BY DENIE

As a result of the processes I have been through and the burning vision within my heart, I know that our inheritance is health, in all its wonderful, glorious, joyful manifestations. Perfect health and vitality is our natural state of being.

Then why is it that record numbers of people are dying of cancer and other degenerative diseases? Why is it that people in the western world are spending more on health-related problems now than in any other time in our history? Why is disease in all its manifestations at an all time high? Why is it that western society is riddled with discontent, emotional dis-empowerment and to most people's reality, financial enslavement? Why is it that the sum total of humanity's experience has left most of the people on this earth, and particularly those living in the western hemisphere, with a sense of abandonment, disconnection from self, and in a state of life-denuding despair? How is it that the greatest industrial achievements this earth has seen, have left our world disharmonious, polluted, toxic and out of step with every aspect of nature? Is this truly what we would call civilization? Is this truly the way we want to live life? Is this in any way "Getting it right?" I suggest not.

I am going to share with you my perception of why we are in this unholy mess and why it is that everywhere I look, I see human beings struggling with their very existence. I will share with you what I perceive as erroneous concepts within our so-called sciences. I will share with you my ideas about how these false perceptions came to be.

I hope you will be able to see a different reality, an electrical reality, a way out of the mire, a way back to life by following your journey to truth and embracing Electrical Nutrition.

Denie Hiestand

VMS, EM, CCI, CL, HbT., Rev.
Vibrational Medicine Specialist, Energy Mastery Certification, Cellelectrology Instructor, Lymphologist, Kinesiologist, Certified Homeobotanical Therapist, Author, Teacher.
International Health Care Professional with a background in Animal Nutrition and over fifteen years in the Human Nutritional field, Founder of the International Academy of Vibrational Medical Science.

INTRODUCTION BY SHELLEY

It has been interesting to watch the incredible responses we have had from readers, especially vegetarians, vegans and others who have realized the value of these concepts, integrated them into their lives and benefited immensely. Being a former vegetarian myself I have experienced how dogmatic I could be in my belief structures, yet my body fell apart after 13 years and I suffered some of "Symptoms of Vegetarianism" outlined in this book. I had six major deficiencies, could no longer participate in vigorous physical activity, was an emotional cot-case, very pale and lethargic, which was definitely not my true nature.

My body has benefited tremendously from understanding its electrical workings, supplementing it with electrically available natural nutritional supplements, drinking electrically alive water, and reintroducing food with nature's electrical matrix that then interfaces seamlessly with my body. I am still very conscious of the source of my food and aim for organic, fresh, mostly raw food and have incorporated good quality animal protein back into my diet. Everybody comments on my vitality, my aliveness, the vibrancy of my complexion and people are amazed at how intense our lifestyle is and what we achieve on a day-to-day basis. *Electrical Nutrition* works!

Denie's revolutionary approach looks at why we as a society have developed so many diseases and illnesses. He takes us beyond normal perceived interpretations and deep into the electrical causes behind the physical manifestations. Denie shares unique hypotheses about the body, why it stops working and how to help it back onto its healing path. He offers the reader profound insights into their own lives and challenges us all to reassess our approach to eating and being. I encourage everyone to read this book at least several times, integrate some of the suggestions and see whether it resonates with you.

Shelley Coleman-Hiestand

LLB (Hons), Reiki Master, Movement and Music Specialist, Vibrational Medicine Researcher. Co-Founder and Facilitator with the International Academy of Vibrational Medical Science.

CHAPTER 1

MYTHS and MEDICAL MISCONCEPTIONS

The fullest expression of the universal life force is what we seek. Anything less than this truth is a state of dis-ease. Now look around you. Can you honestly say that there are many people who exhibit this full expression of life? Do you know anybody who exudes life from every pore of their being? Who is so vibrant and full of energy that they charge the atmosphere of a room when they walk in, or simply make you feel better by being around them? Maybe there are a handful of these healthy, happy souls, but it certainly is not the norm.

This state of vibrant health is our birthright. At our core level, we are vibrant, alive, positive and happy. But, sadly, life's experiences can become a loading on our beingness and the stress of daily existence causes our bodies to degenerate, our emotions to go AWOL and our souls to feel disconnected.

All too often, this is a reality in today's society. But with the information we are sharing, you will be able to make life-affirmative choices, to start to rebuild your physicality and reverse the degenerative process. Once again life will become a joy, a pleasure to be part of.

First, we are going to set out to destroy some of the modern myths and challenge the concepts of how our bodies work; to take what we know and turn it inside out; to look at things differently and to change the parameters of our very thought processes. If, after all this time that humanity has been experiencing this earthly plane of existence, we have only achieved this chronic state of disease and disharmony, then surely it is time we manifested the courage to challenge the premises on which we have based our beliefs.

One erroneous premise that many of our so-called sciences are based upon is that this is a "particle universe." A particle universe is where everything is separate, isolated and disconnected. Science states that the sum total of any equation basically consists of the individual components.

For example, if we take some molecules of hydrogen, which is an explosive gas and one molecule of oxygen, which is the gas required for combustion (burning), you would think, and a particle universe concept would tend to support, that adding them together would make a very big bang and a big fire.

However, quite the opposite happens. When we combine them we make water (H_2O). The combination creates a very different physical and electrical reality than its constituent components. Water is neither explosive nor helpful in the burning process - quite the opposite!

Particle science says one and one makes two, that is, two individual particles added together. But "electrical science" would say that one and one has made "one." Two electrical matrices have combined, changed their electrical construct and are now a completely individual reality with an electrical construct and a physical reality that has no relationship to the original parts. It is now a new and different *singular* whole.

This electrical understanding is not applied to drugs, or their use, in allopathic medicine. It is only now being incorporated into the formulation of some herbal and nutritional supplements (which will be discussed later). Suffice to say that different combinations of drugs, herbs, minerals etc. in different formulations create very different results within the body.

It was 2700 years ago that Thales, the great Greek philosopher, started to philosophize on what the universe was made of (the universal construct). Our science today is still based on his premise that this is an isolationary particle universe. There are no separate particles in the entire cosmos.

Everything, *everything* is made of atoms and atoms are made of *vibrating frequencies of energy*. Energy is everything and everything is energy.

Perhaps we have been going down the wrong path, with the wrong concepts? If the universe is made of energy, then surely we must question current science and its hypotheses. If modern medicine, food production and manufacturing are based on incorrect science, then no wonder we are experiencing ever greater levels of degeneration and disease.

Every single frequency of energy interfaces with, is affected by, and is connected seamlessly, to every other frequency of energy. This is an electrical universe. There is not, there cannot be, there never was and there never will be, an individual, unrelated, anything in this cosmos. There is no separation. All energy is a part of all other energy.

God is light and light is everywhere. The word light derives from the Greek language and in English loosely translates to mean energy. The only way we can understand ourselves, our world and our universe, is to understand it from an energy perspective. The only way we can ever hope to understand our body is from an energy perspective. The only way we can ever alleviate disease is from an energy perspective. The only way to formulate our supplements and our medicine is from an energy perspective. The only way we can make this world into the Garden of Eden is from an energy perspective, because there is nothing else.

By illustrating clearly, in a very logical understandable way, that there is another concept, there is another logic, and in fact there is another premise to our understanding that we can embrace, we will gain the ability to move beyond the boxes of our limited belief structures.

If we are electrical, then this is an electrical universe, and everything we do is an electrical/energetical reality.

If we can achieve this understanding, then everything about our lives - our health, the way we think, feel, process and live as human beings - has the potential to change. To change the concepts that make up our logic, to change the premise that our consciousness is based upon, is to change consciousness itself, and with that our world.

When we become aware of this new premise, that of an electrical universe, and adopt this new consciousness, we will begin to realize just who we are, what we are made of and see the unbelievable joy in this experience called life.

Life can be disease - and pain-free. Life can truly be an experience that we, products of this electrical universe, have a right to experience with total joy.

Having dispatched the concept of the particle universe, we can move onto another of the modern myths - "traditional medicine." Traditional medicine in our western society is often the terminology used to describe our allopathic, or drug-based medical care system. When we look at the word "traditional," according to the Cambridge International Dictionary of English, it means,

"belief, principle or way of acting which people in a particular society or group have continued to follow for a long time...Old/Ancient as in Switzerland has a long tradition of neutrality...tradition as in deeply rooted....a belief followed for a long time without changing, etc., etc."

Therefore, as you can see, to call our present medical system a "traditional" system is one of the greatest misrepresentations of all time.

Our present medical system has only been with us since the early nineteen hundreds. Medical drugs and their use have only come to dominate our health care system in the last thirty years. There is absolutely no long-term history or knowledge pertaining to our modern drug-based medical system. Most of the medical drugs in existence thirty years ago cannot now be used because of their discovered toxic effects.

Our modern allopathic system is the newest, most untried, most unproven, most untraditional health care system in the world. It is the most dangerous experiment in particle science pertaining to chemistry that has ever been foisted upon an unsuspecting populous.

The hijacking of the terminology "traditional medicine" by our health care system is one of history's greatest shams. There is nothing traditional, nothing ancient, nothing steeped in antiquity about any part of our modern health care.

It uses incredibly powerful and toxic substances that the body has no ability to recognize as nutrition, with absolutely no thought given to the electrical bombardment the body suffers as a result of being injected, ingested or exposed to these concoctions.

These chemical compounds hold within them such a disharmonious electrical reality that the body often responds as if an electrical hand grenade had been detonated within. This electrical damage manifests as many different physical symptoms which are medically labelled "side effects." Often these side effects are as devastating or more so than the original problem. Sadly, they sometimes only become apparent years later.

Our so-called medical "professional" seldom informs us of these dangerous and toxic effects prior to recommending these substances. There have been many times in my clinical experience that I have had to deal with major manifestations of these problems, problems as serious as liver and kidney damage and potential failure.

One example springs to mind of a reasonably healthy male, who under a relative degree of stress developed heart burn symptoms. He was prescribed a drug that unbeknown to him had the side effects of causing severe stomach ulceration if taken over a long period.

After three years on this drug, the reasonably healthy man developed severe stomach pain and was eventually diagnosed as having chronic stomach ulcers. The destruction to his stomach was so severe that a succession of five operations resulted in the loss of two thirds of his stomach and intestinal tract.

The resulting lack of digestive ability led to toxic effects throughout his body and he was prescribed more and more drugs to suppress the increasing side effects that developed. This eventually led to kidney and liver damage which became life threatening. Upon investigation by his wife, who researched the available medical literature, she found the originally prescribed drug had severe stomach ulceration listed as a side effect, if prescribed for a period longer than four to six weeks.

Sadly, it is often only when death is a very real possibility that people search for another option. This man was basically knocking on death's door by the time he found his way to my clinic. Suffice to say, the job of rebuilding the electrical function of organs such as the liver and kidneys, is usually not too difficult and in this case was largely achieved.

However, the removal of the toxic residue and the rebuilding of the damaged cells caused by this drug concoction that had been prescribed over many years is a slow and difficult process.

From knocking at death's door, this man is relatively drug free. However, due to the severity of the drug-induced damage to a large part of his system, he will never be a healthy man again. As a result, so-called traditional medicine is now held in contempt by this wonderful family.

Can any of us honestly say that our present medical system, based on toxic substances, is to the overall benefit of the health of humanity? An honest look at the evidence would suggest it is not. However, the incredible amount of knowledge that we have gained as a result of allopathic medicine has certainly created an advantage in specific disease states. The knowledge in organ transplant technology and traumic accident care is without a doubt extremely advantageous and helpful to many people.

There are many thousands of doctors who conscientiously work very diligently not to overprescribe and abuse the power that they have in administering dangerous and toxic drugs.

It would be a wonderful world if all the knowledge from all the known health care systems and modalities were a normal and accepted part of one overall health care system. I fail to see why there is a need for division and antagonistic attitudes between the so-called modalities.

Is not the issue that of assisting the ill person back to a state of health? Surely, the only honest way that assistance can be given is by sharing the benefits of the knowledge that all of humanity has amassed. Sadly, this is seldom the case, and many people do not receive the health care that they should.

A good fifty percent of the clients I have seen in my clinics in the last fifteen years have come to me as a result of medically-induced problems. When all else fails, our present medical system cuts out the malfunctioning part and throws it away, surely suggesting that God got it wrong and taking the attitude that we did not need that bit in the first place. Looking at the "medical misadventures" and the disinformation we are all fed, it is easy to understand that our present medical model must be based on an incorrect premise.

During the ten-year period of the Vietnam war, approximately five thousand (5000) Americans lost their lives per year. Whereas, it has been said, that up to three hundred and sixty thousand (360,000) Americans die **every year** as a result of medical misadventure in American hospitals. These people did not die as the result of the problems they were originally admitted into hospital for, but of other medically and drug induced mistakes/problems.

There was a human outcry over the five thousand per year casualties in Vietnam, and I am astounded by the total lack of voices protesting the devastation to our general populous by the present medical system (experiment).

In a report published by "The Journal of American Medical Association" (JAMA) in the April 14, 1998, issue, by Bruce H. Pomeranz MD, Ph.D., and colleagues from the University of Toronto, it is stated that an estimated 2,216,000 hospital patients experienced a serious ADR each year. The authors define a serious ADR (Adverse Drug Reaction), as one that requires hospitalization, prolongs hospitalization, or one that is permanently disabling or results in death.

Furthermore, they estimate that on the low side ADRs cause more than 106,000 deaths in the United States alone. This makes ADRs between the 4th and 6th largest cause of death in the U.S. And they call it medicine!!!

In another report by Jeffrey A. Johnson and J. Lyle Bootman (from the University of Arizona) published in the Archives of Internal Medicine, vol. 155, October 9, 1995, it is pointed out that preventable illness and death from the misuse of medicines cost the American economy over $75 billion a year. Furthermore, if lost productivity is taken into account, the cost rises to $182 billion.

The researchers point out that the purpose of prescribing pharmaceutical drugs is to treat disease successfully - not to cause more problems. They estimate that this purpose is achieved in less than 40 per cent of all cases. More than 60 percent of all people prescribed pharmaceutical drugs end up with a drug-related problem which results in almost nine million (9,000,000) hospital admissions a year.

As a mater of fact, more that 28 per cent of all hospital admissions in 1992 were due to drug-related illness and somewhere between 80,000 and 200,000 people died from doctor-prescribed medicines.

The researchers conclude that drug-related illness and death should be considered one of the leading "diseases" in the United States.

Another myth many believe in, that our medical system is the best, is sadly just that - a myth. And why? Because our present medical model refuses to even read its own research. The pharmaceutical industry has become so powerful that the knowledge of the electrical understanding of the body and other natural health practices are totally excluded from being available in our "traditional" medical training institutions.

The knowledge of Vibrational Medicine, often called energy healing, has been perfected over thousands of years by many cultures. The healing properties of herbs, botanicals, essential oils, the laying on of hands, the importance of minerals, vitamins etc., has, by and large, been excluded from our current medical paradigm by the enactment of laws. Yet, the most dangerous, life-twisting drugs are injected and ingested with the full backing of these very same laws. And we wonder why we are in this mess.

One of the most basic and oldest forms of one person nurturing another is the beautiful art of massage. The touching of one human by another has profound and measurable effects on all connective (muscle) tissue. There is hardly a mother on this earth who has not massaged her child with gentle loving strokes. There is not a lover who has not given their loved one the same honor.

Yet in many states in the United States of America, there are very tight and restrictive laws that limit and control, and indeed criminalize, its citizens who are not "licensed" to use this most natural and beautiful healing art.

Why? Surely any society that legally controls the honorable touch between two consenting human beings must be a society so screwed up and riddled with undealt with issues that to use the word "civilized" is to border on absurdity.

This is just one example of a pharmaceutical-based medical care system having dictatorial control over governments and, thereby the general public, of anything related to natural health care.

In Polynesian societies, people have been massaging each other for centuries and it is probably the biggest form of nurturing health care in their culture. There are no laws governing two consenting adults gently moving the muscle tissues to assist the flow of oxygen, lymph fluid and health.

Does the enacting of laws in America suggest that we are less able to take responsibility for our own destiny than other cultures? Is the government telling us that we are so stupid that we cannot be trusted to touch each other when and how we see fit? Surely the most natural and basic form of giving somebody something of ourselves - touch - cannot be governed by any overbearing control mechanism.

Apes, chimpanzees and gorillas spend hours touching, massaging and preening each other. In fact, all animals touch and assist each other in their health care. Have we in this society lost so much of our connection to who we are and what health and honor is all about, that we allow ourselves, and in fact encourage, dictatorial control which denies or limits our use of natural healing techniques and remedies?

Take back your power, your right to discern for yourself what is good for you and what is not. This relates also to any of life's circumstances. The move to severely restrict the availability of herbs and other natural health products that have been used by societies for thousands of years must be thwarted.

Any limitation we allow to permeate our lives and our society becomes a limitation of our own life force, which in turn affects each and every cell in our body. The restriction of life force to our cells impacts upon our electrical circuitry with the effect of reducing the flow of energy throughout the body and thus promotes disease.

The Chinese for many centuries have had an understanding of the electrical functions of the body and used this as a basis for a holistic approach to health care.

This electrical knowledge has been taken by some sectors of our modern scientific community to heights never before discovered, yet not one part of this electrical knowledge pertaining to the human body is taught in any of the "traditional" medical learning institutes in North America.

Furthermore, the thousands of years of knowledge that humanity has in the field of herbal medicine is totally denied to us by the same so-called "traditional" medical community. Even the nutritional understanding known in veterinary medicine twenty years ago is still not taught in our medical schools. In fact, until only recently, it was illegal for a doctor in the United States to give basic dietary advice.

Nutrition, in all its forms, is the basis of life. Yet our so-called "health professionals," who are legislated by law to be the guardians of our vitality, had no knowledge, or the legal right, to inform us so we could promote that very vitality. In our folly, we gave our power to this system.

I guess in some ways we get what we deserve, yet my passion for humanity is such that I believe we deserve more.

We deserve the right to all of the knowledge and not just to a legislated section of it that adds to the bottom line profitability of multinational pharmaceutical corporations.

From a health care perspective, we have been fed a large amount of mistruths and disinformation. We have been legislated to accept a health care system that has actually promoted more disharmony, toxic effects and death in the human body than ever before in human history.

It is about time we let go of the myths, falsehoods and disinformation and inform ourselves. It is about time we took responsibility and honored the incredible beings that we are. It is time to take back our power and stop allowing a health care system to desecrate the temples that are our bodies.

Help us get this information out

You can do this by recommending your friends and family to purchase this book, or even buy extra copies and give it to them as presents. We can only continue to do the work and research by having sales of this book. Thank you for supporting us in this manner.

CHAPTER 2

NOURISHMENT - AN ELECTRICAL PROCESS

One of the greatest fallacies most of us believe in, is that **all** food nourishes us. In fact, nothing could be further from the truth.

What is a fact is that everything we eat does one of two things: it either nourishes us or poisons us. The reality is that some (most) of the food we eat actually slowly poisons us. This poisoning starts in our digestive process due to incorrect fermentation.

Fermentation, or digestion, is a Latin-derived word that scientifically describes a very basic process called rotting. In essence, this is all that the stomach component of our digestive tract does - controls the rotting of the food we eat.

To understand, from an electrical perspective, this process called digestion, we need to move beyond a conventional nutritionist's point of view.

To begin with, it is important to realize that the food we eat never ever gets anywhere near the cells in our body. Ninety nine point nine percent of it passes out through our bowels. So, how do we get nourished?

As any farmer or home gardener will tell you, to correctly rot anything you have to match the set of parameters to the different constituent products you are trying to rot.

A farmer making corn silage, which is a carbohydrate, is aware that it requires a different Ph for controlled fermentation than does wet young grass silage, which is a protein. The farmer will often add enzymes and specific bacteria to regulate the Ph for the different food sources about to be fermented.

Our body also needs to change its digestive enzymes and bacteria to regulate the Ph of the digestive juices pertaining to the different types of food about to be digested. This command line is an electrical process.

When we look at a plate of food in front of us, our senses, due to our past experience, recognize what that food is - proteins, carbohydrates, etc. Even before the food gets to our mouth, our body is preparing itself for the coming ingestion. Our visual and smelling senses, then our taste buds and other sensory glands within our mouth cavity, send electrical messages to our digestive tract.

Our stomach responds by excreting the correct substances that change the bacteria and enzymes, thus in turn changes the Ph of our gastric juices. The body changes the fermentation parameters for different foods.

As fermentation can take hours, problems arise when we take one mouthful of potatoes, bread or pasta which are carbohydrates, and the next mouthful we take is of meat, eggs or tofu, which are proteins, or mouthfuls of combinations of carbohydrates and proteins as in a hamburger.

The fermentation of these mouthfuls cannot be carried out correctly because the two substances (protein and carbohydrate) require different fermentation parameters. All compromised fermentation produces toxins. This is the start of all degeneration and disease.

To understand how fermentation works and what this rotting process does to the food to convert it into nourishment, or produce toxins, we need to look at this process in some depth. Keeping it as simple as possible, we will use a lettuce leaf as an example. However all food goes through the same process.

As suggested earlier, most of the food we eat passes out our bowels, meaning it is totally unavailable for our body's nourishment. In essence, the body has no ability to get nourishment from food the way our eyes see it, i.e. physical matter.

Our piece of lettuce, like all vegetation, is predominantly made of cellulose cells, sometimes called roughage or fiber, and the cellulose content of the cells of all vegetation is totally and completely unable to be utilized by the human body.

In fact, most of the world's vegetation is not only unavailable to us as nutrition, but is toxic as well. Our bodies do not relate at all well to the plant kingdom. (It is interesting to note there is not one animal whose flesh is toxic to us.)

The vegetation we commonly refer to as edible food would be more correctly termed "herbs," which is what the edible vegetation used to be called. In times of old, all herbs had medicinal properties and vegetation was largely consumed for these properties and not as the staple diet.

If the lettuce is not available to us as our eyes see it, what happens to the lettuce in order for it to nourish us?

The digestive process starts at our mouth. Humans, not unlike cows, have flat grinding teeth. Also like a cow, we have a jaw that can flex sideways in a grinding motion. It is only the animals on this earth who have a digestive tract capable of fermenting vegetative matter that have this grinding ability. This is because the only part of the lettuce that is going to be available to nourish us is an incredibly small, microscopic component inside the cell of the lettuce.

To extract this single molecule, we first have to use our grinding jaw and teeth structure to fracture and break open the cellulose cell. Then when we swallow, the hopefully very ground up and fractured lettuce will allow the gastric juices, combined with the live enzymes and bacteria that are meant to be in our stomach, to go to work and rapidly break down, or rot (ferment) the previously crushed cellulose structure.

If this fermentation is undertaken correctly, the microscopic molecule will be released from inside the cellulose cell and then be electrically attracted to the field of energy surrounding the cells of the stomach lining. It will then be electrically drawn to and pass through the microscopic pores in the stomach and intestinal lining into the bloodstream.

This microscopic particle is now correctly termed a complex protein molecule and physically has absolutely no relationship to the original lettuce leaf. Ninety nine point nine percent of what started off as our lettuce leaf is now semi-decayed vegetative matter that our body has to get rid of, as there is no further use for it.

The only way the food molecule becomes available to us as nutrition is by this rotting process and as different substances require different parameters to rot correctly, we can see that we have a problem arising from our meat and potato or bread and meat type combinations.

If we take a mouthful of potato, or any carbohydrate, and in the next mouthful we ingest protein, it is not too difficult to see that our stomach will be very confused as to the correct Ph of its gastric juices. In fact, this is exactly what happens...confusion.

There is neither the enzyme nor bacteria balance to create the fermentation that would allow the complete releasing and electrical charging of the protein or the carbohydrate. The breakdown (rotting) from a physical sense could appear to be normal, based on our limited knowledge of nutrition. It is only abnormal when looked at from an electrical perspective.

What actually takes place is the nucleus of the cell is physically released, but its field of energy is somewhat distorted because of the incorrect enzyme, micro bacteria and Ph level. The electrical interface between this stripped molecule and its surrounding environment is not as it should be.

To explain this in a simple way, it would be like trying to start your car with very dirty battery terminals. A small amount of current may flow, but the chances are high that the electrical interface would be slowed or distorted and the engine would not turn over fast enough to start.

This, in effect, is what happens electrically in the stomach. Even though the microscopic nucleus has been released from the cell of the original food, it does not bond itself to the energy surrounding the cells of the stomach lining as it should. Therefore, its progress through to the blood is greatly inhibited or slowed down. Physically we would feel this as a heavy and bloated stomach.

In extreme cases, particularly in a meal containing bread, pasta or potatoes etc. (carbohydrate), and meat, cheese or tofu etc. (protein) [hamburgers are the perfect electrical time bomb], the electrical charge of the molecules would be so out of phase with the field of energy surrounding the cells of the stomach and intestinal tract lining that its electrical disharmony would cause an electrical short circuit in these cells.

When this happens, the natural electrical defenses of these cells start to break down. They then become physically damaged, allowing other decaying matter to seep through the porous lining of the intestinal tract into the blood stream. The result can lead to low-level blood toxicity, low energy levels, hormone imbalances, acne, emotional instability, joint pain, cellulite production (fat) and many other problems in the future.

Furthermore, the damage to the electrical and physical function of the cells in the walls of the intestinal tract can manifest as the disease we call ulcers. The slow destruction of the electrical function of the intestinal lining often leads to the cells' inability to electrically interface with its DNA code. The cells, in essence, lose contact with their instruction manual and then can (and often do) manifest later in life into the disease we call cancer.

Assuming our little food molecule passed through the stomach lining into our blood stream without causing too much electrical disharmony on its way, it would now be called, regardless of its original source (carbohydrate or protein), a protein molecule. The only difference between whether this molecule originated as a carbohydrate or protein food, would be the subtle frequency of energy it contained.

Do not forget this is not food in our normal sense of what food is. We are now talking about a single microscopic molecule that has absolutely no physical resemblance to the original food.

As our blood pumps this molecule around our system, it eventually goes down side roads called capillaries which lead to every cell in our body. These capillaries, when looked at through a microscope, have walls like spider webs. In other words, they are very porous.

However, their holes are of such a size that most of the blood constituent products such as water, bacteria, red blood corpuscles, etc., cannot get through. Some of our tiny little microscopic food particles do get through, while others stay inside the capillaries and deliver their energy via the blood system to the cell.

Those that escape the capillaries enter the lymphatic fluid. This escape is made possible by the electromagnetic field of energy that surrounds the molecular structure of the lymphatic fluid, which is immediately outside of the capillaries. This energy field draws our little food molecule through the gaps in the capillaries, not unlike a magnet drawing iron filings to it.

It is an electrical attraction, an electrical interface, an electrical communication that is taking place. The whole process is so much more in-depth and complicated than our normal nutritional/medical science has ever contemplated.

The journey of our little food molecule from our mouth to our intestinal tract and now to its new home in the lymphatic fluid or the cell, requires possibly up to ten million two way electrical transmissions (communications). **Medical science has little concept of this amazing dance of energy** (or maybe it has chosen not to see this electrical reality?).

Unless the original fermentation or rotting was carried out within the correct parameters, the electrical interchange that was required for this journey would not be completely possible. This disturbance would eventually manifest as physical problems somewhere in our body.

Before there can be any physical "disease," there has to have been an electrical malfunction.

At this stage of our little molecule's journey, what started out as food has not yet been able to release its energy to us. Once the molecule has passed into our lymphatic fluid, something truly amazing happens.

Because of the electrical matrix of the lymphatic fluid, our little molecule is now able to absorb solar or cosmic energy and in fact acts just like a capacitor in an ignition system of some vehicles. It builds up within itself a charge of energy that has the potential to be exponentially far greater than its original charge. However, it still carries within its electrical matrix the original frequency of the food it started out as. In some ways it is not electrically dissimilar to the process of photosynthesis that plants go through.

Plants turn their nutritional uptake into chlorophyll by using sunlight, and this is called photosynthesis. But we are far more evolved and use solar energy to turn our nutrition into powerful sparks of pure energy (advanced photosynthesis?).

The fermentation had to be carried out under the correct parameters and the little molecule's electrical structure cannot be damaged, in order for it to be capable of taking on its full charge of energy. If, however, the fermentation was *not* carried out correctly it would now be electrically *impossible* for our little molecule to become fully charged. This is where the greatest problem for our life force comes about.

The next stage of our electrical nutrition process is that when we move, we pump our lymphatic fluid. As our lymphatic fluid surrounds every cell in our body, our "hopefully fully charged" protein molecule gets moved by the lymphatic fluid and eventually ends up brushing past a cell.

What happens next is the same as lightning. (It is worth mentioning here that there would be no life on earth without lightning.) This process is also identical to a spark plug in your car's gasoline engine, where energy jumps from one polarity to another. Without it, the engine would not be able to function, the fuel (food) would not be used.

As our little molecule's field of energy is of the opposite polarity to that of the cell, it zaps out a spark of energy into the cell and the cell zaps back its spark. Medically, this is called the sodium/potassium pump.

Electrically, this process is an incredibly involved energy transfer. The frequency that was the food has now been discharged into the cell. All of the constituent products that were required by the body from the food have now been transferred ***electrically*** to the body.

The process is totally electrical.

This interchange, this spark of life, contains within it a complexity of which science has very little comprehension of, or understanding. Contained within the spark was the complete matrix of life-giving nutrition that started out as the original food. ***But only if it was fermented correctly.***

From a particle physics point of view, we have no way of explaining this process other than saying that food goes into the body and garbage comes out. From an electrical point of view, an entire consciousness undertakes a change, i.e. the constituent product of the food transforms into the life force of a human being. This is the only way we get nourished. The process is one hundred percent electrical.

This is not a chemical reaction, this is an electrical action.

It could be said that this is the magic of life, the mystery that allows one form of physicality to become another. This, surely, is nature at its supreme evolution.

However, if the original digestion did not take place within the correct parameters for the particular type of food, i.e. protein or carbohydrate, our little molecule would be electrically out of phase on its journey to the lymphatic fluid. All along its journey it would have caused electrical chaos.

Once in the lymphatic fluid, its action would have been similar to a very dirty terminal on a battery. It would not have been able to interface with the lymphatic fluids electrical matrix. Therefore, it would not have been able to achieve its powerful positive charge. Then, when our little molecule brushed past the cell and fired its sodium/potassium pump spark, that spark would have been weak.

This is the point where the electrical matrix of energy contained in the original food would not have been fully available to us. It is at this weak electrical interchange where many of our diseases and degenerative processes start.

After this weak and distorted electrical interchange, our little molecule's field of energy (around the outside of its surface) would not have changed polarity as it was meant to, but would be a mixture of positive and negative, or in other words, electrically dirty. As a result, instead of repulsing its brother and sister molecules, that are also in the lymphatic fluid, our little molecule's electrical disharmony would cause it to attract and to attach itself to its neighbors.

This causes a thick sticky lymphatic fluid, very much harder to move, and as a result we have to go to the gym and do lots of exercise (or receive a good massage) or else we feel sluggish, lethargic and heavy. With movement, the lymphatic system will push our little molecule through thousands of one-way valves called lymph nodes until our molecule ends up at the subclavical valve on each side of our lower neck. At the subclavical valve our little molecule will pass back into the blood stream and from there get delivered to the kidneys.

If its electrical field is out of phase, the kidneys cannot read our molecule as an electrically discharged food particle and promptly send it back to the blood stream instead of into the urinary tract.

Due to its damaged electrical field, our molecule becomes what could be called a "free radical." As a result of this electrical damage, everything this free radical touches becomes electrically damaged.

Consequently, our entire system comes under electrical bombardment. This is why we need to take powerful free radical scavengers, like high dosages of electrically correct vitamin C, vitamin E, and other very high-tech products that are now available (see Appendix).

As well as the free radical damage that is taking place around our body, our little molecule's stickiness now causes globules that our doctor would recognize as cholesterol.

Because our body recognizes these globules as problems within its system, and due to the stickiness brought about by the electrical disharmony, these molecules now attach themselves to the nice clean walls of our blood vessels (the body has to put it somewhere).

It is very easy to see how blocked arteries and angina symptoms begin. Also, these sticky globules end up in our joint cavities and calcify into arthritis and other joint degeneration problems.

The kidneys, in a desperate attempt to clean up the blood, manage to hold onto some of these sticky globules, and we end up with kidney stones. One of the most insidious problems is that some of these globules get pumped around our circulatory system and, because their size is now greater than the size of the openings in the walls of the blood vessels, their escape from the circulatory system is impossible. As a result some of these globules end up in the capillaries (very small diameter blood vessels) and the organ that has the greatest amount of these small diameter capillaries is the brain.

As the sticky globules move into the brain capillaries they eventually get to one where the diameter is smaller than the size of the globule. This sticky mess then blocks the blood flow and the downstream tissues get starved of oxygen and nutrition. These cells can no longer function properly and can die.

Initially, we call this aging. When many capillaries become blocked we start to become concerned about our short term memory, loss of cohesiveness, balance problems and other "aging problems" and say our brain/body is not as good as it used to be. In extreme cases, we have major degenerative diseases like Alzheimers and other motor neuron symptoms developing.

As well as the degenerative diseases that manifest due to years of incorrect food combinations, the damaging process is accentuated by any substance we put into our body that is not electrically available. Food that is not electrically available is any food that has had its natural rotting ability suppressed. This includes foods containing sugar, preservatives, stabilizers and chemicals, plus foods that are packaged, processed, contain artificial flavorings and coloring or have in any way been altered from nature's original electrical matrix.

Remember, it takes approximately ten million electrical messages for an electrically correct food particle to get from our plate to our cells. The slightest interference in this command chain is the initial process of disease. Is it any wonder we are struggling to maintain our health and vitality?

As you can see, the entire modern food handling process, where the emphasis is on long shelf-life, is in fact turning our food into poisons. All processes that limit or slow down the fermentation of food, including pesticides, fungicides, all preservatives, modern food irradiation, including the alteration of the constituent ingredients of natural foods, in fact everything we do to our food, is going to change its electrical function, its electrical matrix, and is going to turn that food into a potential disease-causing time bomb.

The rapid increase in cancer, which is just a highly electrically damaged group of cells, is the almost guaranteed result of supermarket purchased food.

If we index, on a graph, the increase in cancer in our population and superimpose this on a graph showing the increase of manufactured, preserved and chemically-laced foods, those graphs I suggest would resemble each other.

Mother, every time you allow your child to drink a can of pop, to have a cookie, to have some candy, to eat out of a packet of preserved food and eat day after day a predominance of grain-based manufactured foods (breakfast cereal, donuts, pasta and bread, etc.), you are causing within your child's body an electrical time bomb that will be guaranteed to kill it.

Strong words, yes indeed, but nevertheless, sadly, deadly true!

CHAPTER 3

THE ROCK TO ROT THEORY

A great Chinese philosopher has been reported as saying, "First I was a rock, then I was a plant, then I was an animal, and now I am me." Perhaps this little phrase contains the truth of our very existence.

If everything is energy and all energy interfaces with all other energy, this means our body has evolved within the electrical reality pertaining to this dimension. If you like, it had to evolve as part of what we would call nature.

When we look at our nutritional base and follow the chain of nutritional availability backwards, we find that every form of nutrition on this planet originated as inorganic matter. Or, put simply, food on this planet started out as a rock. All our nutrition comes from this source.

A rock also consists of vibrating frequencies of energy (very slow vibrating frequencies), so in that sense it is alive. However, the vibratory rate of a rock is such that its constituent nutritional components are unavailable to us directly.

Let us look at life forms as a scale. At one end of this scale we have very low frequency forms of life called rocks and at the opposite end of this scale we have humans, the highest vibratory rate life form. Looking at this evolution from a nutritional point of view, every life form between these two extremes has an important and naturally structured place in the increasing vibratory rate scale, from the inorganic rock to the flesh and bones that make up our bodies.

Looking at it another way, the lowest form of life on this planet is that which does not rot, a rock. That which is the most evolved away from the rock, the highest vibratory rate, is that which decays the most rapidly, such as flesh. From an electrical nutrition viewpoint, the higher the vibration of the foods we eat, the greater the life force available to us.

The rocks, which consists of inorganic compounds have in them every known mineral needed for our nourishment. At the frequency of a rock, the compounds and minerals are physically and electrically unavailable to us. We would die eating rocks.

Next in the food chain are the micro organisms that live on and gnaw into the rock and in fact start the entire process of food availability. The lichen and other fungus come next, living on the remains and the nutrients that the micro organisms extracted from the rocks. The lichen and fungus digest and refine these nutrients one stage further in their digestive tract and the nutrients then become their life.

Next come the micro bacteria that create the food in the soil for the small plants. The roots of the plants take up the nutrients left behind by the decaying lichen, fungus and bacteria. Within the soil there are still more micro bacteria, eating, digesting and dying, refining the original nutrients still further into available food for the plants.

The plants evolve this food one more step, increase their vibratory rate one more notch and thus this food becomes the plant's body. Plants, as science will tell us, are higher in vibratory rate than rocks.

As the vibratory rate of this evolving life form increases, its physicality moves away from that of a rock. Or put another way, a rock does not decay, but plant material does.

Then along comes the animal, eats the plant and refines its constituent products even further. The vibratory rate is increased even more and what started out as a rock, becomes a plant and is now bounding around as an animal. Animal flesh decays much faster than plant life.

Once again, we have a demonstration that shows us that as life evolves, life force increases, as evidenced by an increase in vibratory rate that can be measured as an increase in rotting ability. Thus, the further we evolve away from the rock, the less like it we become, the quicker we rot. Science would call this evolution.

We humans then come along and eat the animals and take that evolutionary stage one step further. The animal then becomes our life which is the highest vibratory rate form on this planet. We can prove this premise with the rock to rot theory because human flesh is known to be the fastest decaying flesh of all.

Therefore, from a nutritional point of view, to supply ourselves with the highest vibratory rate food possible, the best choice would be human flesh. Perhaps this is why human sacrifice was part of many of our known ancient cultures (*The Power of Myth*, by Joseph Campbell). In fact, the person selected for these sacrificial festivals, was none other than the most succulent, vibrant, pure young girl at the start of her puberty, who would be the highest in the evolutionary chain and thus contain the most life force.

The fact that a young woman was always chosen is because the vibratory rate of a female is greater than that of a male - the female species is actually more evolved from an electrical perspective. The selection of the young maiden and the ingestion of her flesh had the most profound effect on the vitality and vibrancy of the remaining tribal group who partook. That is why it was considered an honor, the highest honor, the greatest possible gift one could ever give to their tribal group, that of their very essence, their life.

Some ancient cultures were also known to eat human flesh as a part of their diet. This is referred to as cannibalism. Some tribes in times of famine would sacrifice a small number of themselves to ensure the survival of the whole.

Perhaps the often-murmured phrase from a mother to her child of "I just love you so much, I could gobble you all up," and the lovers feeling of, "I just want to take you and eat you, you're so yummy," are very real expressions of a deep energy truth. At some level we are obviously aware of the profound effect to our life force when we become one with another.

It could be seen as a strange concept that our society expresses feelings of horror about human sacrifice, yet still allows and in fact encourages our young to go to war. War is all about destruction and control of others. Sacrifice, in the context of our discussion with regard to the ancient cultures, was about enhancing life, not destroying it. It was about honor and giving, not manipulation and taking.

Following is a account that demonstrates the unbelievable nutrition-giving ability of the highest evolved life force on this planet, us.

A number of years back, a small plane, loaded with a senior high school football team, crashed in the mountains of South America. A number of the young men survived the crash, but because of the damage to the plane and its radio equipment they were not able to communicate their survival to the outside world and the search parties never found them.

Given up for dead and facing starvation, the only food source available to them was the very well preserved frozen bodies of their dead teammates. Naturally, starvation soon drove them to the realization that any food was better than nothing. And so began their ingestion of the raw flesh of their fellow humans.

After some time of waiting, they realized that rescue was not an option, so two of the strongest elected to attempt to walk to civilization. They sun dried some human flesh to take with them. Remember, this was the only food they had available: no grains, no vegetables, no fruit, nothing, only human flesh.

The walk took the two young men a number of weeks. In the process they crossed several mountain ranges and some of the most rugged terrain in the world. They walked from daylight to dark in all weather. Eventually, they reached a village and the rescue of their friends was undertaken.

When the medical authorities checked the young men's health, they were amazed at their physical condition. The most astounding part of this whole story is that when the authorities calculated the calories the two young men would have used in their incredible physical feat to get out of the mountains, the amount of meat they had with them could not have supplied the calorific value that would have been required.

However, the calorific value was calculated from what animal protein would have supplied. It appeared the human flesh supplied to the boys three times the energy value than would have been expected. They were in amazingly good health. There were no nutritional deficiencies.

However, ingesting human flesh is not now socially acceptable, therefore the next best source of nourishment would be one step down the vibratory ladder, to that of the animal kingdom.

Obviously these electrical nutrition and frequency increase concepts open up a whole new argument with regards to the vegetarian way of nutrition that has become popular in the last ten to twenty years in the Western world.

CHAPTER 4

VEGETARIANS' ELECTRICAL NON-SENSE

One basis for vegetarianism is that animal products are a lower life form and contain a lower frequency of energy than the plant kingdom. If we look at the vibratory rate of animal flesh as compared to that of vegetation, in terms of the "rock to rot" theory, we find this to be a totally erroneous concept.

Another of the vegetarians' arguments for not ingesting animal flesh is that the fear the animal feels when being slaughtered remains within the electrical matrix of the flesh. This is a possibility; however in reality, different animals react differently in the slaughtering process.

A hunted animal, hunted with reverence and honor will offer itself and thus will carry no traumatic frequencies. Domestic cattle and sheep - even in the slaughterhouse scenario - show no emotional reaction. On the other hand, hogs will display extreme emotional fear in that same slaughterhouse environment.

Commercially produced chicken are totally traumatized at all times due to their unbelievably cramped and overcrowded cages, and react with extreme fear when slaughtered. The most disharmonious food by far, from an electrical point of view, would be battery farmed chicken (nearly all supermarket and fast food chicken is from this source).

All slaughtering undertaken with honor and as part of a ceremonial sacrifice, as in halal killing practised in the Middle East and Kosher slaughtering in Israel and other ceremonies practised by many cultures around the world, balances many of the emotional traumatic frequencies that one would be concerned about. That is why previous cultures slaughtered with ceremony.

Today in New Zealand and Australia, there are tens of thousands of sheep slaughtered in the slaughter houses with individual ceremonial ritual and prayers of thanks for each animal, given by the attending holy person.

This is carried out so that these animals can be exported to countries which require slaughtering in the presence of a holy person. Also, this is the reasoning behind the Christian ritual of saying grace before the food is consumed. The fact of honoring the food and its source has a powerful effect on normalizing any disharmonic frequencies contained within it.

From an energy perspective, the vegetarian concept of not wanting to eat meat because it entails killing is also based on an erroneous paradigm. It would be difficult indeed, actually impossible, to live on this earth without killing.

With every breath we take, we ingest and kill countless millions of microscopic bacteria that live in the air. Every time we wash our hands, it has been said, we kill approximately three million individual life forms, commonly referred to as bacteria, and just imagine the wholesale destruction of life every time we take a shower! And what about when we put our feet on the ground? Once again we are killing millions of life forms (squish!).

So you see, everything we do, everything we touch, every breath we take, we are in the killing business. This earth plane existence of ours is all about one life form becoming another. In essence there is no death, there is only a changing of frequency.

I chuckle to myself when vegetarians tell me that they do not eat meat because they do not want to kill an animal, yet they will quite happily eat spirulina, which is in essence thousands of microscopic "critters." (Blue/green algae are sometimes referred to as "animal" due to their likeness in many aspects to the animal kingdom. Also its flesh is protein, and algae are definitely very much alive.)

So what are we saying here? It is okay to kill if we can not see it? To me, that is like the little child hiding in the corner with its hands covering its eyes thinking nobody can see it! My suggestion is, it is about time a lot of folk got their logic straight.

Everything contains a consciousness, everything is a vibrating frequency of energy, everything is alive. When you take a carrot from the ground, are you not separating it from what was its life? When you cut the lettuce from its stem, are you not separating it from its life? In fact, there is quite a well known scientific experiment that shows the frequency of energy contained within a carrot has a bigger change when pulled from the ground than a cattle beast's energy changes when slaughtered.

It could be said that the carrot actually screams louder than the cow. Just as the slaughtering of an animal needs to be done with reverence and honor, so too do we need to take the vegetables with the same reverence and honor.

It is not the slaughtering and ingesting that is the issue, but rather the honor we give to the process.

Everything is alive and the only way anything survives in this dimension is by taking the vibratory rate of another and absorbing it as part of self. Nothing survives, nothing lives, without this ingestion of something else that is alive.

The theory that vegetables are better for you because they are alive, and that animal flesh is not good for you because it is dead, is once again based on a totally incorrect premise. Aliveness, as we have demonstrated, can only be quantified by its vibratory rate, the frequency that is contained within its cellular structure.

This vibratory rate is reflected in the amount of time it takes for a substance to decay. Life is not only measured by whether something is running around or not. On that premise, all fruit and vegetables are dead, which shows the idiocy of that thought process. The less life force there is, the slower it decays. The more life force there is, the quicker it decays.

We can make choices of which food will give us the most life-giving nutrition and the biggest evolutionary gain. To perceive any natural food, food that evolved as part of nature, that contains nature's electrical matrix, as dead, is to have an extremely limited and distorted understanding of what nutrition, and in fact life, is.

It is important also to understand the agricultural process so we can make informed choices regarding which proteins we ingest.

When different animal raising techniques are compared, it always shocks me that some consumers in the supermarket will purchase commercially raised chicken in the belief that they are getting a healthier product than red meat. In reality, nothing could be further from the truth. The chicken industry simply won the propaganda war.

Commercial chicken farming is usually a highly sophisticated, extremely regimented battery farming operation. The birds are caged and fed an artificially formulated diet that sometimes contains, as a normal ingredient, antibiotics. The antibiotic content of the food ration is often required on an ongoing basis due to the crammed cages and chronic disease potential of the battery farming regime.

Modern hens have been genetically bred to have an astonishingly fast growth rate for a few weeks. They are slaughtered at this very young age before chronic disease has time to manifest. However, at this stage the hen has never seen sunlight and due to its forced growth its flesh is extremely anaemic. It in no way carries within it the correct electrical matrix that would give us the nutrition we would expect. This is a very different animal than what grandma served up for Sunday roast when we were kids.

Buying our lovely packaged chicken from the supermarket, we could be getting an electrically distorted, genetically altered, hormone induced tender, force-fed, antibiotic-laced, deficient form of protein. But it looks nice.

Another misconception is that red meat, particularly beef, contains high levels of antibiotics and hormones. Once again it is important to be educated so that we can make informed choices. There is too much misinformation and lack of knowledge by the general consumer, particularly in North America, regarding red meat.

A cattle beast starts off its life foraging on the range country, or in outside feedlots. It stays with its mother for approximately six to nine months and then is weaned onto grass if it is in the range country, or onto alfalfa hay and corn silage if it is a feedlot-reared calf. The range cattle, at approximately three hundred days of age, will be brought into the feedlot and then fed the same diet as the feedlot-reared stock for another hundred days or so.

At approximately four hundred days of age, this cattle beast is regarded as prime. It is now slaughtered and that is what ends up at your restaurants and supermarkets as prime cuts, steaks, etc. This meat is practically hormone-free, antibiotic free, and unaltered in any way.

A young cattle beast is an incredibly hardy animal and, unlike commercially produced chickens, cattle beasts are raised outside. Their feed consists of either range grass or in the case of the feed lots, top quality alfalfa hay and corn silage, both of which require far less chemicals in their production than wheat or barley (the normal feed stock for chickens).

Our beef cattle finishing industry, which produces our prime beef, is at the top end of the food production squeaky clean scale. However, the manufactured beef (beef that goes into the ground beef hamburger, sausages and beef products other than the prime cuts), is made up of some different classes of animals.

The dairy herd, which are housed lactating animals, are machine milked twice a day and this can make them very susceptible to udder infections, necessitating the need for antibiotic treatment if an infection develops. However, the milk from an antibiotic treated cow is never intentionally supplied to the milk factory because the milk is tested daily and the penalties are extremely severe.

Dairy cows are at times fed with a natural hormone to increase their milk production. This increases her hormone and milk levels only fractionally due to the physical constraints of her udder capacity. Farmers are not stupid, to over stimulate a cows milk production would be detrimental to her health and thereby the farmers profitability (I know, I was a dairy farmer for many years).

Antibiotics and hormones can stay in the flesh of the cow for some time, but when the dairy cow has finished its life as a milk producing animal its meat is graded "manufacturing" not "prime" and this manufacturing grade meat goes to the ground beef market. Bull beef is also used in the ground beef manufacturing process because its water retention properties are required for the meat patties.

Farming bulls is a difficult and dangerous occupation, and to stay alive and have the farm's fences, equipment and buildings all in one piece, the farmer is sometimes required to use hormonal treatments to quieten the bulls down. Bulls are big, wild, strong animals! The hormone used is like the one naturally produced in the females (cows). This makes the bulls behave more like the females, i.e. much easier to handle.

Understanding how agriculture works and looking at the commercially available meat sources, it would be a fair comment to state that as far as the meats produced in North America go, prime red meat is probably one of the cleanest, most environmentally pure and nutritious forms of protein available. One of the readily available sources of meat of this quality is the prime beef that carries the "Angus Beef" certification/trademark. Ground beef would be down a grade or two. The hormone and antibiotic use in the dairy and beef industry is way lower than most people surmize.

Farming is all about having healthy animals. There is no profitability in having sick cows that need medication. Northwest salmon would be right up there with prime red meat. There are not many people in the arctic Pacific throwing chemicals and toxins around.

Commercially produced chicken would be at the other end of the scale, along with U.S. hog meat. A large proportion of what Americans see in their supermarkets as hog meat, and especially bacon, would be condemned to the blood and bone fertilizer plants in most other western countries. Most Americans do not know what quality bacon looks like.

Hog farmers in the U.S. get paid per pound of live weight. The more the animal weighs, the more the farmers get paid. By comparison, in Canada, New Zealand, Australia and England, the farmers get severely financially penalized if their hogs weigh over a certain figure. They are also penalized if the percentage of fat is over the allowable limit, and every hog is tested electronically for its fat coverage. Quality gets rewarded and quantity gets penalized. In the U.S. the opposite seems to be the case.

Correctly graded lamb from New Zealand or Australia would be even better than some prime beef, as these animals never see anything except their mothers' milk, natural green grass and the joy of life. Sadly, it is difficult to purchase genuine lamb (which is a young sheep less than nine months of age) in the continental U.S.A.

The grading system for sheep meat in the U.S. often does not distinguish between young and old sheep. When you purchase U.S. "lamb," it could be an old ewe (old female sheep with meat as tough as old boots and a smell to fit). Everywhere else in the world this would be graded as mutton.

Real "lamb" is a specifically defined age and weight specification that can be relied upon if sourced from New Zealand or Australia. It is arguably the purest and environmentally cleanest meat source produced anywhere in the world.

Looking at other forms of protein, nuts are extremely valuable and readily available, but miss some of the B group vitamins and amino acids that red meat has. However on the rock to rot scale nuts do not fare too well, as they are very slow to rot. Peanuts remember, are not nuts, they are not protein, they are tubers, carbohydrates like potatoes.

Another popular protein source in our modern culture is spirulina (blue/green algae). It is easily digested and quickly assimilated. Spirulina is an excellent alternative or additional source of amino acids, B group vitamins and absorbable iron (especially good for menstruating women and breast feeding mothers). Be aware of the source of your spirulina. Search out an organically produced product as this will be more electrically available to your body.

Tofu, another protein source, is made from soya beans and is one of the most highly processed electrically damaged forms of protein we could possibly eat. Its manufacturing requires the stripping and recombining of the molecular structure of the soya bean.

The electrical matrix of commercial tofu is completely and utterly foreign to our bodies. Homemade naturally fermented tofu may be more electrically available. However, nature does not produce tofu, therefore tofu does not contain nature's electrical matrix. In my opinion, tofu, as a healthy protein option, is extremely suspect when looked at from an electrical nutrition point of view.

There are a number of published papers on different trials that support this. A major investigation on the health of long term tofu eaters was undertaken in Japan with three thousand five hundred participants and completed in 1998.

The result of this trial was that tofu eaters had far greater health problems than the control group. Overwhelmingly, it demonstrated the onset of serious degenerative diseases much earlier in life in the tofu eating group, Alzheimers being one of the main problems. This trial brought to the attention of the health authorities that the incidence of Alzheimers in this group was the highest of any group in Japan. *Note soy info on Pg 58.*

This trial supports the electrical nutrition concept that any food that does not contain nature's electrical matrix will cause serious degenerative problems, sooner rather than later.

Similarly, juicing fruits and vegetables also dramatically alters the electrical matrix and no longer provides food as nature intended. I have personally seen the results of toxic effects developing when someone overdoses on juiced vegetables in the belief that they were living very healthily. Take care, your digestive tract was never intended to absorb excessive amounts of twentieth century juicing technology.

Sometimes, too much juicing results in diarrhea, which is a symptom of an extremely stressed and agitated digestive tract, not a desirable state to be in.

However, in severe life-threatening dis-ease states, such as cancer and liver failure, juicing would be advantageous due to the fact that the cellulose of the cell walls of the food would be fractured, therefore making the food molecules more easily accessible to the body. This has the effect of lowering the energy required for digestion and that energy could then be used to assist the body in its recovery process.

If you know where you can procure free range, organically grown chickens or any other certified organic meats, go for it! The same applies to any other organically produced food. The certification of organically produced products is now well established and highly integrous.

Expect to pay more for good clean food, because in every way, including its electrical availability, it is by far the best choice. The organic farmers themselves know what harmonious production of food is all about. Organic farming is often more a lifestyle choice and not necessarily a commercial operation. Pay them well for their beautiful life giving products - they have earned it.

As a result of many questions we have been asked since the original publication of *Electrical Nutrition,* regarding statements in the preceding pages that Tofu and Soy are extremely toxic to the body, in this edition we present to you a tremendous amount of science pertaining to the whole "Soya" issue. As Denie often says in his public presentations, as far as agriculture is concerned, Soy has always been toxic to animals and was never used as a food, only as a ground conditioner, ie. it inoculates nitrogen into the soil. The following report is printed with the kind and grateful permission of Sally Fallon & Mary G. Enig, PhD (with attached endnotes). This report backs up, from a scientific point of view, precisely what Denie has been saying from an electrical stand point. Soy and Tofu are toxic, always have been and always will be. But we will leave you, the reader, to decide and you can make your choices from a much more informed basis after you have read the following:

Tragedy and Hype
The Third International Soy Symposium

Far from being the perfect food, modern soy products contain antinutrients and toxins and they interfere with the absorption of vitamins and minerals.

Each year, research on the health effects of soy and soybean components seems to increase exponentially. Furthermore, research is not just expanding in the primary areas under investigation, such as cancer, heart disease and osteoporosis; new findings suggest that soy has potential benefits that may be more extensive than previously thought.

So writes Mark Messina, PhD, General Chairperson of the Third International Soy Symposium, held in Washington, DC, in November 1999.[1] For four days, well-funded scientists gathered in Washington made presentations to an admiring press and to their sponsors - United Soybean Board, American Soybean Association, Monsanto, Protein Technologies International, Central Soya, Cargill Foods, Personal Products Company, SoyLife, Whitehall-Robins Healthcare and the soybean councils of Illinois, Indiana, Kentucky, Michigan, Minnesota, Nebraska, Ohio and South Dakota.

The symposium marked the apogee of a decade-long marketing campaign to gain consumer acceptance of tofu, soy milk, soy ice cream, soy cheese, soy sausage and soy derivatives, particularly soy isoflavones like genistein and diadzen, the oestrogen-like compounds found in soybeans. It coincided with a US Food and Drug Administration (FDA) decision, announced on October 25, 1999, to allow a health claim for products "low in saturated fat and cholesterol" that contain 6.25 grams of soy protein per serving. Breakfast cereals, baked goods, convenience food, smoothie mixes and meat substitutes could now be sold with labels touting benefits to cardiovascular health, as long as these products contained one heaping teaspoon of soy protein per 100-gram serving.

MARKETING THE PERFECT FOOD

"Just imagine you could grow the perfect food. This food not only would provide affordable nutrition, but also would be delicious and easy to prepare in a variety of ways. It would be a healthful food, with no saturated fat. In fact, you would be growing a virtual fountain of youth on your back forty." The author is Dean Houghton, writing for The Furrow,[2] a magazine published in 12 languages by John Deere. "This ideal food would help prevent, and perhaps reverse, some of the world's most dreaded diseases. You could grow this miracle crop in a variety of soils and climates. Its cultivation would build up, not deplete, the land...this miracle food already exists... It's called soy."

Just imagine. Farmers have been imagining - and planting more soy. What was once a minor crop, listed in the 1913 US Department of Agriculture (USDA) handbook not as a food but as an industrial product, now covers 72 million acres of American farmland. Much of this harvest will be used to feed chickens, turkeys, pigs, cows and salmon. Another large fraction will be squeezed to produce oil for margarine, shortenings and salad dressings.

Advances in technology make it possible to produce isolated soy protein from what was once considered a waste product - the defatted, high-protein soy chips - and then transform something that looks and smells terrible into products that can be consumed by human beings. Flavorings, preservatives, sweeteners, emulsifiers and synthetic nutrients have turned soy protein isolate, the food processors' ugly duckling, into a New Age Cinderella.

The new fairy-tale food has been marketed not so much for her beauty but for her virtues. Early on, products based on soy protein isolate were sold as extenders and meat substitutes - a strategy that failed to produce the requisite consumer demand. The industry changed its approach. "The quickest way to gain product acceptability in the less affluent society," said an industry spokesman, "is to have the product consumed on its own merit in a more affluent society."[3] So soy is now sold to the upscale consumer, not as a cheap, poverty food but as a miracle substance that will prevent heart disease and cancer, whisk away hot flushes, build strong bones and keep us forever young. The competition - meat, milk, cheese, butter and eggs - has been duly demonized by the appropriate government bodies. Soy serves as meat and milk for a new generation of virtuous vegetarians.

Marketing costs money, especially when it needs to be bolstered with "research," but there's plenty of funds available. All soybean producers pay a mandatory assessment of one-half to one per cent of the net market price of soybeans. The total - something like US$80 million annually[4] - supports United Soybean's program to "strengthen the position of soybeans in the marketplace and maintain and expand domestic and foreign markets for uses for soybeans and soybean products".

State soybean councils from Maryland, Nebraska, Delaware, Arkansas, Virginia, North Dakota and Michigan provide another $2.5 million for "research."[5] Private companies like Archer Daniels Midland also contribute their share. ADM spent $4.7 million for advertising on Meet the Press and $4.3 million on Face the Nation during the course of a year.[6] Public relations firms help convert research projects into newspaper articles and advertising copy, and law firms lobby for favorable government regulations. IMF money funds soy processing plants in foreign countries, and free trade policies keep soybean abundance flowing to overseas destinations.

The push for more soy has been relentless and global in its reach. Soy protein is now found in most supermarket breads. It is being used to transform "the humble tortilla, Mexico's corn-based staple food, into a protein-fortified 'super-tortilla' that would give a nutritional boost to the nearly 20 million Mexicans who live in extreme poverty."[7] Advertising for a new soy-enriched loaf from Allied Bakeries in Britain targets menopausal women seeking relief from hot flushes. Sales are running at a quarter of a million loaves per week.[8]

The soy industry hired Norman Robert Associates, a public relations firm, to "get more soy products onto school menus."[9] The USDA responded with a proposal to scrap the 30 per cent limit for soy in school lunches. The NuMenu program would allow unlimited use of soy in student meals. With soy added to hamburgers, tacos and lasagna, dieticians can get the total fat content below 30 per cent of calories, thereby conforming to government dictates. "With the soy-enhanced food items, students are receiving better servings of nutrients and less cholesterol and fat."

Soy milk has posted the biggest gains, soaring from $2 million in 1980 to $300 million in the US last year.[10] Recent advances in processing have transformed the grey, thin, bitter, beany-tasting Asian beverage into a product that Western consumers will accept - one that tastes like a milkshake, but without the guilt.

Processing miracles, good packaging, massive advertising and a marketing strategy that stresses the products' possible health benefits account for increasing sales to all age groups. For example, reports that soy helps prevent prostate cancer have made soy milk acceptable to middle-aged men. "You don't have to twist the arm of a 55- to 60-year-old guy to get him to try soy milk," says Mark Messina. Michael Milken, former junk bond financier, has helped the industry shed its hippie image with well-publicized efforts to consume 40 grams of soy protein daily.

America today, tomorrow the world. Soy milk sales are rising in Canada, even though soy milk there costs twice as much as cow's milk. Soybean milk processing plants are sprouting up in places like Kenya.[11] Even China, where soy really is a poverty food and whose people want more meat, not tofu, has opted to build Western-style soy factories rather than develop western grasslands for grazing animals.[12]

CINDERELLA'S DARK SIDE

The propaganda that has created the soy sales miracle is all the more remarkable because, only a few decades ago, the soybean was considered unfit to eat - even in Asia. During the Chou Dynasty (1134 - 246 BC) the soybean was designated one of the five sacred grains, along with barley, wheat, millet and rice. However, the pictograph for the soybean, which dates from earlier times, indicates that it was not first used as a food; for whereas the pictographs for the other four grains show the seed and stem structure of the plant, the pictograph for the soybean emphasizes the root structure. Agricultural literature of the period speaks frequently of the soybean and its use in crop rotation. Apparently the soy plant was initially used as a method of fixing nitrogen.[13]

The soybean did not serve as a food until the discovery of fermentation techniques, some time during the Chou Dynasty. The first soy foods were fermented products like tempeh, natto, miso and soy sauce. At a later date, possibly in the 2nd century BC, Chinese scientists discovered that a purée of cooked soybeans could be precipitated with calcium sulphate or magnesium sulphate (plaster of Paris or Epsom salts) to make a smooth, pale curd - tofu or bean curd. The use of fermented and precipitated soy products soon spread to other parts of the Orient, notably Japan and Indonesia.

The Chinese did not eat unfermented soybeans as they did other legumes such as lentils because the soybean contains large quantities of natural toxins or "antinutrients." First among them are potent enzyme inhibitors that block the action of trypsin and other enzymes needed for protein digestion. These inhibitors are large, tightly folded proteins that are not completely deactivated during ordinary cooking. They can produce serious gastric distress, reduced protein digestion and chronic deficiencies in amino acid uptake. In test animals, diets high in trypsin inhibitors cause enlargement and pathological conditions of the pancreas, including cancer.[14]

Soybeans also contain haemaglutinin, a clot-promoting substance that causes red blood cells to clump together.

Trypsin inhibitors and haemaglutinin are growth inhibitors. Weanling rats fed soy containing these antinutrients fail to grow normally. Growth-depressant compounds are deactivated during the process of fermentation, so once the Chinese discovered how to ferment the soybean, they began to incorporate soy foods into their diets. In precipitated products, enzyme inhibitors concentrate in the soaking liquid rather than in the curd. Thus, in tofu and bean curd, growth depressants are reduced in quantity but not completely eliminated.

Soy also contains goitrogens - substances that depress thyroid function.

Soybeans are high in phytic acid, present in the bran or hulls of all seeds. It's a substance that can block the uptake of essential minerals - calcium, magnesium, copper, iron and especially zinc - in the intestinal tract. Although not a household word, phytic acid has been extensively studied; there are literally hundreds of articles on the effects of phytic acid in the current scientific literature. Scientists are in general agreement that grain- and legume-based diets high in phytates contribute to widespread mineral deficiencies in third world countries.[15] Analysis shows that calcium, magnesium, iron and zinc are present in the plant foods eaten in these areas, but the high phytate content of soy- and grain-based diets prevents their absorption.

The soybean has one of the highest phytate levels of any grain or legume that has been studied[16] and the phytates in soy are highly resistant to normal phytate-reducing techniques such as long, slow cooking.[17] Only a long period of fermentation will significantly reduce the phytate content of soybeans. When precipitated soy products like tofu are consumed with meat, the mineral-blocking effects of the phytates are reduced.[18] The Japanese traditionally eat a small amount of tofu or miso as part of a mineral-rich fish broth, followed by a serving of meat or fish.

Vegetarians who consume tofu and bean curd as a substitute for meat and dairy products risk severe mineral deficiencies. The results of calcium, magnesium and iron deficiency are well known; those of zinc are less so.

Zinc is called the intelligence mineral because it is needed for optimal development and functioning of the brain and nervous system. It plays a role in protein synthesis and collagen formation; it is involved in the blood-sugar control mechanism and thus protects against diabetes; it is needed for a healthy reproductive system. Zinc is a key component in numerous vital enzymes and plays a role in the immune system. Phytates found in soy products interfere with zinc absorption more completely than with other minerals.[19] Zinc deficiency can cause a "spacey" feeling that some vegetarians may mistake for the "high" of spiritual enlightenment.

Milk drinking is given as the reason why second-generation Japanese in America grow taller than their native ancestors. Some investigators postulate that the reduced phytate content of the American diet - whatever may be its other deficiencies - is the true explanation, pointing out that both Asian and Western children who do not get enough meat and fish products to counteract the effects of a high phytate diet, frequently suffer rickets, stunting and other growth problems.[20]

SOY PROTEIN ISOLATE: NOT SO FRIENDLY

Soy processors have worked hard to get these antinutrients out of the finished product, particularly soy protein isolate (SPI) which is the key ingredient in most soy foods that imitate meat and dairy products, including baby formulas and some brands of soy milk.

SPI is not something you can make in your own kitchen. Production takes place in industrial factories where a slurry of soy beans is first mixed with an alkaline solution to remove fiber, then precipitated and separated using an acid wash and, finally, neutralized in an alkaline solution. Acid washing in aluminum tanks leaches high levels of aluminum into the final product. The resultant curds are spray-dried at high temperatures to produce a high-protein powder. A final indignity to the original soybean is high-temperature, high-pressure extrusion processing of soy protein isolate to produce textured vegetable protein (TVP).

Much of the trypsin inhibitor content can be removed through high-temperature processing, but not all. Trypsin inhibitor content of soy protein isolate can vary as much as fivefold.[21] (In rats, even low-level trypsin inhibitor SPI feeding results in reduced weight gain compared to controls.[22]) But high-temperature processing has the unfortunate side-effect of so denaturing the other proteins in soy that they are rendered largely ineffective.[23] That's why animals on soy feed need lysine supplements for normal growth.

Nitrites, which are potent carcinogens, are formed during spray-drying, and a toxin called lysinoalanine is formed during alkaline processing.[24] Numerous artificial flavorings, particularly MSG, are added to soy protein isolate and textured vegetable protein products to mask their strong "beany" taste and to impart the flavor of meat.[25]

In feeding experiments, the use of SPI increased requirements for vitamins E, K, D and B12 and created deficiency symptoms of calcium, magnesium, manganese, molybdenum, copper, iron and zinc.[26] Phytic acid remaining in these soy products greatly inhibits zinc and iron absorption; test animals fed SPI develop enlarged organs, particularly the pancreas and thyroid gland, and increased deposition of fatty acids in the liver.[27]

Yet soy protein isolate and textured vegetable protein are used extensively in school lunch programs, commercial baked goods, diet beverages and fast food products. They are heavily promoted in third world countries and form the basis of many food giveaway programs.

In spite of poor results in animal feeding trials, the soy industry has sponsored a number of studies designed to show that soy protein products can be used in human diets as a replacement for traditional foods. An example is "Nutritional Quality of Soy Bean Protein Isolates: Studies in Children of Preschool Age," sponsored by the Ralston Purina Company.[28]

A group of Central American children suffering from malnutrition was first stabilized and brought into better health by feeding them native foods, including meat and dairy products. Then, for a two-week period, these traditional foods were replaced by a drink made of soy protein isolate and sugar. All nitrogen taken in and all nitrogen excreted was measured in truly Orwellian fashion: the children were weighed naked every morning, and all excrement and vomit gathered up for analysis. The researchers found that the children retained nitrogen and that their growth was "adequate," so the experiment was declared a success.

Whether the children were actually healthy on such a diet, or could remain so over a long period, is another matter. The researchers noted that the children vomited "occasionally," usually after finishing a meal; that over half suffered from periods of moderate diarrhea; that some had upper respiratory infections; and that others suffered from rash and fever.

It should be noted that the researchers did not dare to use soy products to help the children recover from malnutrition, and were obliged to supplement the soy-sugar mixture with nutrients largely absent in soy products - notably, vitamins A, D and B12, iron, iodine and zinc.

FDA HEALTH CLAIM CHALLENGED

The best marketing strategy for a product that is inherently unhealthy is, of course, a health claim.

"The road to FDA approval," writes a soy apologist, "was long and demanding, consisting of a detailed review of human clinical data collected from more than 40 scientific studies conducted over the last 20 years. Soy protein was found to be one of the rare foods that had sufficient scientific evidence not only to qualify for an FDA health claim proposal but to ultimately pass the rigorous approval process."[29]

The "long and demanding" road to FDA approval actually took a few unexpected turns. The original petition, submitted by Protein Technology International, requested a health claim for isoflavones, the oestrogen-like compounds found plentifully in soybeans, based on assertions that "only soy protein that has been processed in a manner in which isoflavones are retained will result in cholesterol lowering." In 1998, the FDA made the unprecedented move of rewriting PTI's petition, removing any reference to the phyto-estrogens and substituting a claim for soy protein - a move that was in direct contradiction to the agency's regulations. The FDA is authorized to make rulings only on substances presented by petition.

The abrupt change in direction was no doubt due to the fact that a number of researchers, including scientists employed by the US Government, submitted documents indicating that isoflavones are toxic.

The FDA had also received, early in 1998, the final British Government report on phyto-estrogens, which failed to find much evidence of benefit and warned against potential adverse effects.[30]

Even with the change to soy protein isolate, FDA bureaucrats engaged in the "rigorous approval process" were forced to deal nimbly with concerns about mineral blocking effects, enzyme inhibitors, goitrogenicity, endocrine disruption, reproductive problems and increased allergic reactions from consumption of soy products.[31]

One of the strongest letters of protest came from Dr Dan Sheehan and Dr Daniel Doerge, government researchers at the National Center for Toxicological Research.[32] *Their pleas for warning labels were dismissed as unwarranted.*

"Sufficient scientific evidence" of soy's cholesterol-lowering properties is drawn largely from a 1995 meta-analysis by Dr James Anderson, sponsored by Protein Technologies International and published in the New England Journal of Medicine.[33]

A meta-analysis is a review and summary of the results of many clinical studies on the same subject. Use of meta-analyses to draw general conclusions has come under sharp criticism by members of the scientific community. "Researchers substituting meta-analysis for more rigorous trials risk making faulty assumptions and indulging in creative accounting," says Sir John Scott, President of the Royal Society of New Zealand. "Like is not being lumped with like. Little lumps and big lumps of data are being gathered together by various groups."[34]

There is the added temptation for researchers, particularly researchers funded by a company like Protein Technologies International, to leave out studies that would prevent the desired conclusions. Dr Anderson discarded eight studies for various reasons, leaving a remainder of twenty-nine. The published report suggested that individuals with cholesterol levels over 250 mg/dl would experience a "significant" reduction of 7 to 20 per cent in levels of serum cholesterol if they substituted soy protein for animal protein. Cholesterol reduction was insignificant for individuals whose cholesterol was lower than 250 mg/dl.

In other words, for most of us, giving up steak and eating veggie burgers instead will not bring down blood cholesterol levels. The health claim that the FDA approved "after detailed review of human clinical data" fails to inform the consumer about these important details.

Research that ties soy to positive effects on cholesterol levels is "incredibly immature," said Ronald M. Krauss, MD, head of *the Molecular Medical Research Program and Lawrence Berkeley National Laboratory.[35] He might have added that studies in which cholesterol levels were lowered through either diet or drugs have consistently resulted in a greater number of deaths in the treatment groups than in controls - deaths from stroke, cancer, intestinal disorders, accident and suicide.[36] Cholesterol-lowering measures in the US have fuelled a $60 billion per year cholesterol-lowering industry, but have not saved us from the ravages of heart disease.*

SOY AND CANCER

The new FDA ruling does not allow any claims about cancer prevention on food packages, but that has not restrained the industry and its marketeers from making them in their promotional literature.

"In addition to protecting the heart," says a vitamin company brochure, "soy has demonstrated powerful anticancer benefits...the Japanese, who eat 30 times as much soy as North Americans, have a lower incidence of cancers of the breast, uterus and prostate."[37]

Indeed they do. But the Japanese, and Asians in general, have much higher rates of other types of cancer, particularly cancer of the esophagus, stomach, pancreas and liver.[38] Asians throughout the world also have high rates of thyroid cancer.[39] The logic that links low rates of reproductive cancers to soy consumption requires attribution of high rates of thyroid and digestive cancers to the same foods, particularly as soy causes these types of cancers in laboratory rats.

Just how much soy do Asians eat? A 1998 survey found that the average daily amount of soy protein consumed in Japan was about eight grams for men and seven for women - less than two teaspoons.[40] The famous Cornell China Study, conducted by Colin T. Campbell, found that legume consumption in China varied from 0 to 58 grams per day, with a mean of about twelve.[41] Assuming that two-thirds of legume consumption is soy, then the maximum consumption is about 40 grams, or less than three tablespoons per day, with an average consumption of about nine grams, or less than two teaspoons. A survey conducted in the 1930s found that soy foods accounted for only 1.5 per cent of calories in the Chinese diet, compared with 65 per cent of calories from pork.[42] *(Asians traditionally cooked with lard, not vegetable oil!)*

Traditionally fermented soy products make a delicious, natural seasoning that may supply important nutritional factors in the Asian diet. But except in times of famine, Asians consume soy products only in small amounts, as condiments, and not as a replacement for animal foods - with one exception. Celibate monks living in monasteries and leading a vegetarian lifestyle find soy foods quite helpful because they dampen libido.

It was a 1994 meta-analysis by Mark Messina, published in Nutrition and Cancer, that fuelled speculation on soy's anticarcinogenic properties.[43] *Messina noted that in 26 animal studies, 65 per cent reported protective effects from soy. He conveniently neglected to include at least one study in which soy feeding caused pancreatic cancer - the 1985 study by Rackis.*[44]

In the human studies he listed, the results were mixed. A few showed some protective effect, but most showed no correlation at all between soy consumption and cancer rates. He concluded that "the data in this review cannot be used as a basis for claiming that soy intake decreases cancer risk." Yet in his subsequent book, The Simple Soybean and Your Health, Messina makes just such a claim, recommending one cup or 230 grams of soy products per day in his "optimal" diet as a way to prevent cancer.

Thousands of women are now consuming soy in the belief that it protects them against breast cancer. Yet, in 1996, researchers found that women consuming soy protein isolate had an increased incidence of epithelial hyperplasia, a condition that presages malignancies.[45] *A year later, dietary genistein was found to stimulate breast cells to enter the cell cycle - a discovery that led the study authors to conclude that women should not consume soy products to prevent breast cancer.*[46]

PHYTOESTROGENS: PANACEA OR POISON?

The male species of tropical birds carries the drab plumage of the female at birth and 'colors up' at maturity, somewhere between nine and 24 months.

In 1991, Richard and Valerie James, bird breeders in Whangerei, New Zealand, purchased a new kind of feed for their birds - one based largely on soy protein.[47] When soy-based feed was used, their birds 'colored up' after just a few months. In fact, one bird-food manufacturer claimed that this early development was an advantage imparted by the feed. A 1992 ad for Roudybush feed formula showed a picture of the male crimson rosella, an Australian parrot that acquires beautiful red plumage at 18 to 24 months, already brightly colored at 11 weeks old.

Unfortunately, in the ensuing years, there was decreased fertility in the birds, with precocious maturation, deformed, stunted and stillborn babies, and premature deaths, especially among females, with the result that the total population in the aviaries went into steady decline. The birds suffered beak and bone deformities, goiter, immune system disorders and pathological, aggressive behavior. Autopsy revealed digestive organs in a state of disintegration. The list of problems corresponded with many of the problems the James's had encountered in their two children, who had been fed soy-based infant formula.

Startled, aghast, angry, the James's hired toxicologist Mike Fitzpatrick. PhD, to investigate further. Dr Fitzpatrick's literature review uncovered evidence that soy consumption has been linked to numerous disorders, including infertility, increased cancer and infantile leukemia; and, in studies dating back to the 1950s,[48] that genistein in soy causes endocrine disruption in animals. Dr Fitzpatrick also analyzed the bird feed and found that it contained high levels of phyto-estrogens, especially genistein. When the James's discontinued using soy-based feed, the flock gradually returned to normal breeding habits and behavior.

The James's embarked on a private crusade to warn the public and government officials about toxins in soy foods, particularly the endocrine-disrupting isoflavones, genistein and diadzen. Protein Technology International received their material in 1994.

In 1991, Japanese researchers reported that consumption of as little as 30 grams or two tablespoons of soybeans per day for only one month resulted in a significant increase in thyroid-stimulating hormone.[49] Diffuse goiter and hypothyroidism appeared in some of the subjects and many complained of constipation, fatigue and lethargy, even though their intake of iodine was adequate. In 1997, researchers from the FDA's National Center for Toxicological Research made the embarrassing discovery that the goitrogenic components of soy were the very same isoflavones.[50]

Twenty-five grams of soy protein isolate, the minimum amount PTI claimed to have cholesterol-lowering effects, contains from 50 to 70 mg of isoflavones. It took only 45 mg of isoflavones in pre-menopausal women to exert significant biological effects, including a reduction in hormones needed for adequate thyroid function. These effects lingered for three months after soy consumption was discontinued.[51]

One hundred grams of soy protein - the maximum suggested cholesterol-lowering dose, and the amount recommended by Protein Technologies International - can contain almost 600 mg of isoflavones[52] an amount that is undeniably toxic. In 1992, the Swiss health service estimated that 100 grams of soy protein provided the estrogenic equivalent of the Pill.[53]

In vitro studies suggest that isoflavones inhibit synthesis of estradiol and other steroid hormones.[54] Reproductive problems, infertility, thyroid disease and liver disease due to dietary intake of isoflavones have been observed for several species of animals including mice, cheetah, quail, pigs, rats, sturgeon and sheep.[55]

It is the isoflavones in soy that are said to have a favorable effect on postmenopausal symptoms, including hot flushes, and protection from osteoporosis. Quantification of discomfort from hot flushes is extremely subjective, and most studies show that control subjects report reduction in discomfort in amounts equal to subjects given soy.[56] The claim that soy prevents osteoporosis is extraordinary, given that soy foods block calcium and cause vitamin D deficiencies. If Asians indeed have lower rates of osteoporosis than Westerners, it is because their diet provides plenty of vitamin D from shrimp, lard and seafood, and plenty of calcium from bone broths. The reason that Westerners have such high rates of osteoporosis is because they have substituted soy oil for butter, which is a traditional source of vitamin D and other fat-soluble activators needed for calcium absorption.

BIRTH CONTROL PILLS FOR BABIES

But it was the isoflavones in infant formula that gave the James's the most cause for concern. In 1998, investigators reported that the daily exposure of infants to isoflavones in soy infant formula is 6 to 10 times higher on a body-weight basis than the dose that has hormonal effects in adults consuming soy foods. Circulating concentrations of isoflavones in infants fed soy-based formula were 13,000 to 22,000 times higher than plasma estradiol concentrations in infants on cow's milk formula.[57]

Approximately 25 per cent of bottle-fed children in the US receive soy-based formula - a much higher percentage than in other parts of the Western world. Fitzpatrick estimated that an infant exclusively fed soy formula receives the estrogenic equivalent (based on body weight) of at least five birth control pills per day.[58] *By contrast, almost no phyto-estrogens have been detected in dairy-based infant formula or in human milk, even when the mother consumes soy products.*

Scientists have known for years that soy-based formula can cause thyroid problems in babies. But what are the effects of soy products on the hormonal development of the infant, both male and female?

Male infants undergo a "testosterone surge" during the first few months of life, when testosterone levels may be as high as those of an adult male. During this period, the infant is programmed to express male characteristics after puberty, not only in the development of his sexual organs and other masculine physical traits, but also in setting patterns in the brain characteristic of male behavior. In monkeys, deficiency of male hormones impairs the development of spatial perception (which, in humans, is normally more acute in men than in women), of learning ability and of visual discrimination tasks (such as would be required for reading).[59] *It goes without saying that future patterns of sexual orientation may also be influenced by the early hormonal environment. Male children exposed during gestation to diethylstilbestrol (DES), a synthetic oestrogen that has effects on animals similar to those of phyto-estrogens from soy, had testes smaller than normal on maturation.*[60]

Learning disabilities, especially in male children, have reached epidemic proportions. Soy infant feeding - which began in earnest in the early 1970s - cannot be ignored as a probable cause for these tragic developments.

As for girls, an alarming number are entering puberty much earlier than normal, according to a recent study reported in the journal Pediatrics.[61] Investigators found that one per cent of all girls now show signs of puberty, such as breast development or pubic hair, before the age of three; by age eight, 14.7 per cent of white girls and almost 50 per cent of African-American girls have one or both of these characteristics.

New data indicate that environmental estrogens such as PCBs and DDE (a breakdown product of DDT) may cause early sexual development in girls.[62] In the 1986 Puerto Rico Premature Thelarche study, the most significant dietary association with premature sexual development was not chicken - as reported in the press - but soy infant formula.[63]

The consequences of this truncated childhood are tragic. Young girls with mature bodies must cope with feelings and urges that most children are not well-equipped to handle. And early maturation in girls is frequently a harbinger for problems with the reproductive system later in life, including failure to menstruate, infertility and breast cancer.

Parents who have contacted the James's recount other problems associated with children of both sexes who were fed soy-based formula, including extreme emotional behavior, asthma, immune system problems, pituitary insufficiency, thyroid disorders and irritable bowel syndrome - the same endocrine and digestive havoc that afflicted the James' parrots.

DISSENSION IN THE RANKS

Organizers of the Third International Soy Symposium would be hard-pressed to call the conference an unqualified success. On the second day of the symposium, the London-based Food Commission and the Weston A. Price Foundation of Washington, DC, held a joint press conference, in the same hotel as the symposium, to present concerns about soy infant formula. Industry representatives sat stony-faced through the recitation of potential dangers and a plea from concerned scientists and parents to pull soy-based infant formula from the market. Under pressure from the James's, the New Zealand Government had issued a health warning about soy infant formula in 1998; it was time for the American government to do the same.

On the last day of the symposium, presentations on new findings related to toxicity sent a well-oxygenated chill through the giddy helium hype. Dr. Lon White reported on a study of Japanese Americans living in Hawaii, that showed a significant statistical relationship between two or more servings of tofu a week and "accelerated brain aging." [64] Those participants who consumed tofu in mid-life had lower cognitive function in late life and a greater incidence of Alzheimer's disease and dementia. "What's more," said Dr White, "those who ate a lot of tofu, by the time they were 75 or 80 looked five years older"[65] White and his colleagues blamed the negative effects on isoflavones - a finding that supports an earlier study in which postmenopausal women with higher levels of circulating oestrogen experienced greater cognitive decline.[66]

Scientists Daniel Sheehan and Daniel Doerge, from the National Center for Toxicological Research, ruined PTI's day by presenting findings from rat feeding studies, indicating that genistein in soy foods causes irreversible damage to enzymes that synthesize thyroid hormones.[67] "The association between soybean consumption and goiter in animals and humans has a long history," wrote Dr Doerge. "Current evidence for the beneficial effects of soy requires a full understanding of potential adverse effects as well."

Dr Claude Hughes reported that rats born to mothers that were fed genistein had decreased birth weights compared to controls, and onset of puberty occurred earlier in male offspring.[68] His research suggested that the effects observed in rats "...will be at least somewhat predictive of what occurs in humans. There is no reason to assume that there will be gross malformations of fetuses but there may be subtle changes, such as neurobehavioral attributes, immune function and sex hormone levels." The results, he said, "could be nothing or could be something of great concern...if mom is eating something that can act like sex hormones, it is logical to wonder if that could change the baby's development."[69]

A study of babies born to vegetarian mothers, published in January 2000, indicated just what those changes in baby's development might be. Mothers who ate a vegetarian diet during pregnancy had a fivefold greater risk of delivering a boy with hypospadias, a birth defect of the penis.[70] The authors of the study suggested that the cause was greater exposure to phyto-estrogens in soy foods popular with vegetarians. Problems with female offspring of vegetarian mothers are more likely to show up later in life. While soy's estrogenic effect is less than that of diethylstilbestrol (DES), the dose is likely to be higher because it's consumed as a food, not taken as a drug. Daughters of women who took DES during pregnancy suffered from infertility and cancer when they reached their twenties.

QUESTION MARKS OVER GRAS STATUS

Lurking in the background of industry hype for soy is the nagging question of whether it's even legal to add soy protein isolate to food. All food additives not in common use prior to 1958, including casein protein from milk, must have GRAS (Generally Recognized As Safe) status. In 1972, the Nixon administration directed a re-examination of substances believed to be GRAS, in the light of any scientific information then available. This re-examination included casein protein which became codified as GRAS in 1978. In 1974, the FDA obtained a literature review of soy protein because, as soy protein had not been used in food until 1959 and was not even in common use in the early 1970s, it was not eligible to have its GRAS status grand fathered under the provisions of the Food, Drug and Cosmetic Act.[71]

The scientific literature up to 1974 recognized many antinutrients in factory-made soy protein, including trypsin inhibitors, phytic acid and genistein. But the FDA literature review dismissed discussion of adverse impacts, with the statement that *it was important for "adequate processing" to remove them. Genistein could be removed with an alcohol wash, but it was an expensive procedure that processors avoided. Later studies determined that trypsin inhibitor content could be removed only with long periods of heat and pressure, but the FDA has imposed no requirements for manufacturers to do so.*

The FDA was more concerned with toxins formed during processing, specifically nitrites and lysinoalanine.[72] Even at low levels of consumption - averaging one-third of a gram per day at the time - the presence of these carcinogens was considered too great a threat to public health to allow GRAS status.

Soy protein did have approval for use as a binder in cardboard boxes, and this approval was allowed to continue, as researchers considered that migration of nitrites from the box into the food contents would be too small to constitute a cancer risk. FDA officials called for safety specifications and monitoring procedures before granting of GRAS status for food. These were never performed. To this day, use of soy protein is codified as GRAS only for this limited industrial use as a cardboard binder. This means that soy protein must be subject to premarket approval procedures each time manufacturers intend to use it as a food or add it to a food.

Soy protein was introduced into infant formula in the early 1960s. It was a new product with no history of any use at all. As soy protein did not have GRAS status, premarket approval was required. This was not and still has not been granted. The key ingredient of soy infant formula is not recognized as safe.

THE NEXT ASBESTOS?

"Against the backdrop of widespread praise...there is growing suspicion that soy - despite its undisputed benefits - may pose some health hazards," writes Marian Burros, a leading food writer for the New York Times. More than any other writer, Ms Burros's endorsement of a low-fat, largely vegetarian diet has herded Americans into supermarket aisles featuring soy foods.

Yet her January 26, 2000 article, "Doubts Cloud Rosy News on Soy," contains the following alarming statement: "Not one of the 18 scientists interviewed for this column was willing to say that taking isoflavones was risk free." Ms Burros did not enumerate the risks, nor did she mention that the recommended 25 daily grams of soy protein contain enough isoflavones to cause problems in sensitive individuals, but it was evident that the industry had recognized the need to cover itself.

Because the industry is extremely exposed...contingency lawyers will soon discover that the number of potential plaintiffs can be counted in the millions and the pockets are very, very deep. Juries will hear something like the following: "The industry has known for years that soy contains many toxins. At first they told the public that the toxins were removed by processing. When it became apparent that processing could not get rid of them, they claimed that these substances were beneficial. Your government granted a health claim to a substance that is poisonous, and the industry lied to the public to sell more soy."

The "industry" includes merchants, manufacturers, scientists, publicists, bureaucrats, former bond financiers, food writers, vitamin companies and retail stores. Farmers will probably escape because they were duped like the rest of us. But they need to find something else to grow before the soy bubble bursts and the market collapses: grass-fed livestock, designer vegetables...or hemp to make paper for thousands and thousands of legal briefs.

Endnotes:

1. *Program for the Third International Symposium on the Role of Soy in Preventing and Treating Chronic Disease, Sunday, October 31, through Wednesday, November 3, 1999, Omni Shoreham Hotel, Washington, DC.*

2. *Houghton, Dean, "Healthful Harvest", The Furrow, January 2000, pp. 10-13.*

3. *Coleman, Richard J., "Vegetable Protein - A Delayed Birth?" Journal of the American Oil Chemists' Society 52:238A, April 1975.*

4. *See www/unitedsoybean.org.*

5. *These are listed in www.soyonlineservice.co.nz.*

6. *Wall Street Journal, October 27, 1995.*

7. Smith, James F., "Healthier tortillas could lead to healthier Mexico", Denver Post, August 22, 1999, p. 26A.

8. "Bakery says new loaf can help reduce hot flushes", Reuters, September 15, 1997.

9. "Beefing Up Burgers with Soy Products at School", Nutrition Week, Community Nutrition Institute, Washington, DC, June 5, 1998, p. 2.

10. Urquhart, John, "A Health Food Hits Big Time", Wall Street Journal, August 3, 1999, p. B1

11. "Soyabean Milk Plant in Kenya", Africa News Service, September 1998.

12. Simoons, Frederick J., Food in China: A Cultural and Historical Inquiry, CRC Press, Boca Raton, 1991, p. 64.

13. Katz, Solomon H., "Food and Biocultural Evolution: A Model for the Investigation of Modern Nutritional Problems", Nutritional Anthropology, Alan R. Liss Inc., 1987, p. 50.

14. Rackis, Joseph J. et al., "The USDA trypsin inhibitor study. I. Background, objectives and procedural details", Qualification of Plant Foods in Human Nutrition, vol. 35, 1985.

15. Van Rensburg et al., "Nutritional status of African populations predisposed to esophageal cancer", Nutrition and Cancer, vol. 4, 1983, pp. 206-216; Moser, P.B. et al., "Copper, iron, zinc and selenium dietary intake and status of Nepalese lactating women and their breastfed infants", American Journal of Clinical Nutrition 47:729-734, April 1988; Harland, B.F. et al., "Nutritional status and phytate: zinc and phytate X calcium: zinc dietary molar ratios of lacto-ovovegetarian Trappist monks: 10 years later", Journal of the American Dietetic Association 88:1562-1566, December 1988.

16. El Tiney, A.H., "Proximate Composition and Mineral and Phytate Contents of Legumes Grown in Sudan", Journal of Food Composition and Analysis (1989) 2:6778.

17. Ologhobo, A.D. et al., "Distribution of phosphorus and phytate in some Nigerian varieties of legumes and some effects of processing", Journal of Food Science 49(1):199-201, January/ February 1984.

18. Sandstrom, B. et al., "Effect of protein level and protein source on zinc absorption in humans", Journal of Nutrition 119(1):48-53, January 1989; Tait, Susan et al., "The availability of minerals in food, with particular reference to iron", Journal of Research in Society and Health 103(2):74-77, April 1983.

19. Phytate reduction of zinc absorption has been demonstrated in numerous studies. These results are summarized in Leviton, Richard, Tofu, Tempeh, Miso and Other Soyfoods: The 'Food of the Future' - How to Enjoy Its Spectacular Health Benefits, Keats Publishing, Inc., New Canaan, CT, USA, 1982, p. 1415.

20. Mellanby, Edward, "Experimental rickets: The effect of cereals and their interaction with other factors of diet and environment in producing rickets", Journal of the Medical Research Council 93:265, March 1925; Wills, M.R. et al., "Phytic Acid and Nutritional Rickets in Immigrants", The Lancet, April 8,1972, pp. 771-773.

21. Rackis et al., ibid.

22. Rackis et al., ibid., p. 232.

23. Wallace, G.M., "Studies on the Processing and Properties of Soymilk", Journal of Science and Food Agriculture 22:526-535, October 1971.

24. Rackis, et al., ibid., p. 22; "Evaluation of the Health Aspects of Soy Protein Isolates as Food Ingredients", prepared for FDA by Life Sciences Research Office, Federation of American Societies for Experimental Biology (9650 Rockville Pike, Bethesda, MD 20014), USA, Contract No. FDA 223-75-2004, 1979.

25. See www/truthinlabeling.org.

26. Rackis, Joseph, J., "Biological and Physiological Factors in Soybeans", Journal of the American Oil Chemists' Society 51:161A-170A, January 1974.

27. Rackis, Joseph J. et al., "The USDA trypsin inhibitor study", ibid.

28. Torum, Benjamin, "Nutritional Quality of Soybean Protein Isolates: Studies in Children of Preschool Age", in Soy Protein and Human Nutrition, Harold L Wilcke et al. (eds), Academic

Press, New York, 1979.

29. Zreik, Marwin, CCN, "The Great Soy Protein Awakening", Total Health 32(1), February 2000.

30. IEH Assessment on Phyto-estrogens in the Human Diet, Final Report to the Ministry of Agriculture, Fisheries and Food, UK, November 1997, p. 11.

31. Food Labeling: Health Claims: Soy Protein and Coronary Heart Disease, Food and Drug Administration 21 CFR, Part 101 (Docket No. 98P-0683).

32. Sheegan, Daniel M. and Daniel R Doerge, Letter to Dockets Management Branch (HFA-305), February 18, 1999.

33. Anderson, James W. et al., "Meta-analysis of the Effects of Soy Protein Intake on Serum Lipids", New England Journal of Medicine (1995) 333:(5):276-282.

34. Guy, Camille, "Doctors warned against magic, quackery", New Zealand Herald, September 9, 1995, section 8, p. 5.

35. Sander, Kate and Hilary Wilson, "FDA approves new health claim for soy, but little fallout expected for dairy", Cheese Market News, October 22, 1999, p. 24.

36. Enig, Mary G. and Sally Fallon, "The Oiling of America", NEXUS Magazine, December 1998-January 1999 and February-March 1999; also available at www.WestonAPrice.org.

37. Natural Medicine News (L & H Vitamins, 32-33 47th Avenue, Long Island City, NY 11101), USA, January/February 2000, p. 8.

38. Harras, Angela (ed.), Cancer Rates and Risks, National Institutes of Health, National Cancer Institute, 1996, 4th edition.

39. Searle, Charles E. (ed.), Chemical Carcinogens, ACS Monograph 173, American Chemical Society, Washington, DC, 1976.

40. Nagata, C. et al., Journal of Nutrition (1998) 128:209-213.

41. Campbell, Colin T. et al., The Cornell Project in China.

42. Chang, K.C. (ed.), Food in Chinese Culture: Anthropological and Historical Perspectives, New Haven, 1977.

43. Messina, Mark J. et al., "Soy Intake and Cancer Risk: A Review of the In Vitro and In Vivo Data", Nutrition and Cancer (1994) 21(2):113-131.

44. Rackis et al, "The USDA trypsin inhibitor study", ibid.

45. Petrakis, N.L. et al., "Stimulatory influence of soy protein isolate on breast secretion in pre- and post-menopausal women", Cancer Epid. Bio. Prev. (1996) 5:785-794.

46. Dees, C. et al., "Dietary estrogens stimulate human breast cells to enter the cell cycle", Environmental Health Perspectives (1997) 105(Suppl. 3):633-636.

47. Woodhams, D.J., "Phyto-estrogens and parrots: The anatomy of an investigation", Proceedings of the Nutrition Society of New Zealand (1995) 20:22-30.

48. Matrone, G. et al., "Effect of Genistin on Growth and Development of the Male Mouse", Journal of Nutrition (1956) 235-240.

49. Ishizuki, Y. et al., "The effects on the thyroid gland of soybeans administered experimentally in healthy subjects", Nippon Naibunpi Gakkai Zasshi (1991) 767:622-629.

50. Divi, R.L. et al., "Anti-thyroid isoflavones from the soybean", Biochemical Pharmacology (1997) 54:1087-1096.

51. Cassidy, A. et al., "Biological Effects of a Diet of Soy Protein Rich in Isoflavones on the Menstrual Cycle of Pre-menopausal Women", American Journal of Clinical Nutrition (1994) 60:333-340.

52. Murphy, P.A., "Phytoestrogen Content of Processed Soybean Foods", Food Technology, January 1982, pp. 60-64.

53. Bulletin de L'Office Fédéral de la Santé Publique, no. 28, July 20, 1992.

54. Keung, W.M., "Dietary estrogenic isoflavones are potent inhibitors of B-hydroxysteroid dehydrogenase of P. testosteronii", Biochemical and Biophysical Research Committee (1995)

215:1137-1144; Makela, S.I. et al., "Estrogen-specific 12 B-hydroxysteroid oxidoreductase type 1 (E.C. 1.1.1.62) as a possible target for the action of phyto-estrogens", PSEBM (1995) 208:51-59.

55. Setchell, K.D.R. et al., "Dietary estrogens - a probable cause of infertility and liver disease in captive cheetahs", Gastroenterology (1987) 93:225-233; Leopald, A.S., "Phyto-estrogens: Adverse effects on reproduction in California Quail," Science (1976) 191:98-100; Drane, H.M. et al., "Estrogenic activity of soya-bean products", Food, Cosmetics and Technology (1980) 18:425-427; Kimura, S. et al., "Development of malignant goiter by defatted soybean with iodine-free diet in rats", Gann. (1976) 67:763-765; Pelissero, C. et al., "Estrogenic effect of dietary soybean meal on vitellogenesis in cultured Siberian Sturgeon Acipenser baeri", Gen. Comp. End. (1991) 83:447-457; Braden et al., "The estrogenic activity and metabolism of certain isoflavones in sheep", Australian J. Agricultural Research (1967) 18:335-348.

56. Ginsburg, Jean and Giordana M. Prelevic, "Is there a proven place for phyto-estrogens in the menopause?", Climacteric (1999) 2:75-78.

57. Setchell, K.D. et al., "Isoflavone content of infant formulas and the metabolic fate of these early phyto-estrogens in early life", American Journal of Clinical Nutrition, December 1998 Supplement, 1453S-1461S.

58. Irvine, C. et al., "The Potential Adverse Effects of Soybean Phyto-estrogens in Infant Feeding", New Zealand Medical Journal May 24, 1995, p. 318.

59. Hagger, C. and J. Bachevalier, "Visual habit formation in 3-month-old monkeys (Macaca mulatta): reversal of sex difference following neonatal manipulations of androgen", Behavior and Brain Research (1991) 45:57-63.

60. Ross, R.K. et al., "Effect of in-utero exposure to diethylstilbestrol on age at onset of puberty and on post-pubertal hormone levels in boys", Canadian Medical Association Journal 128(10):1197-8, May 15, 1983.

61. Herman-Giddens, Marcia E. et al., "Secondary Sexual Characteristics and Menses in Young Girls Seen in Office Practice: A Study from the Pediatric Research in Office Settings Network", Pediatrics 99(4):505-512, April 1997.

62. Rachel's Environment & Health Weekly 263, "The Wingspread Statement", Part 1, December 11, 1991; Colborn, Theo, Dianne Dumanoski and John Peterson Myers, Our Stolen Future, Little, Brown & Company, London, 1996.

63. Freni-Titulaer, L.W., "Premature Thelarch in Puerto Rico: A search for environmental factors", American Journal of Diseases of Children 140(12):1263-1267, December 1986.

64. White, Lon, "Association of High Midlife Tofu Consumption with Accelerated Brain Aging", Plenary Session #8: Cognitive Function, The Third International Soy Symposium, November 1999, Program, p. 26.

65. Altonn, Helen, "Too much tofu induces 'brain aging', study shows", Honolulu Star-Bulletin, November 19, 1999.

66. Journal of the American Geriatric Society (1998) 46:816-21.

67. Doerge, Daniel R., "Inactivation of Thyroid Peroxidase by Genistein and Daidzein in Vitro and in Vivo; Mechanism for Anti-Thyroid Activity of Soy", presented at the November 1999 Soy Symposium in Washington, DC, National Center for Toxicological Research, Jefferson, AR 72029, USA.

68. Hughes, Claude, Center for Women's Health and Department of Obstetrics & Gynecology, Cedars-Sinai Medical Center, Los Angeles, CA.

69. Soy Intake May Affect Fetus", Reuters News Service, November 5, 1999.

70. "Vegetarian diet in pregnancy linked to birth defect", BJU International 85:107-113, January 2000.

71. FDA ref 72/104, Report FDABF GRAS - 258.

72. *"Evaluation of the Health Aspects of Soy Protein Isolates as Food Ingredients", prepared for FDA by Life Sciences Research Office, Federation of American Societies for Experimental Biology (FASEB) (9650 Rockville Pike, Bethesda, MD 20014, USA), Contract No, FDA 223-75-2004, 1979.*

About the Authors:

Sally Fallon is the author of Nourishing Traditions: The Cookbook that Challenges Politically Correct Nutrition and the Diet Dictocrats (1999, 2nd edition, New Trends Publishing, tel +1 877 707 1776 or +1 219 268 2601) and President of the Weston A. Price Foundation, Washington, DC (www.WestonAPrice.org).

Mary G. Enig, PhD, is the author of Know Your Fats: The Complete Primer for Understanding the Nutrition of Fats, Oils and Cholesterol (2000, Bethesda Press, www.BethesdaPress.com), is President of the Maryland Nutritionists Association and Vice President of the Weston A. Price Foundation, Washington, DC.

The authors wish to thank Mike Fitzpatrick, PhD, and Valerie and Richard James for their help in preparing this article.

The authors of Electrical Nutrition wish to thank all of the above for this article and permission to include it in this book.

Help us get this information out

You can do this by recommending your friends and family to purchase this book, or even buy extra copies and give it to them as presents. We can only continue to do the work and research by having sales of this book. Thank you for supporting us in this manner.

CHAPTER 5

SYMPTOMS OF VEGETARIANISM

The greatest travesty I see in my clinical work is that of the vegetarian community and their overall malnourishment. It is frighteningly clear to me every time an ardent vegetarian walks into my clinic. I have literally hundreds of former vegetarians on my client base. In fact, when young women come to me with reproductive system problems that have usually manifested in their inability to conceive, my stock response is "If you are ardent in your desire to maintain your vegetarian diet, you will have difficulty in keeping your body working." The reason is that I would be only treating the symptom(s) and not the cause. The cause could well be malnutrition with severe protein deficiency.

Protein deficiency, amino acid and mineral depletion coupled with chronic low levels of vitality are rampant among the vegetarians of the western hemisphere. My clinical experience is that ninety percent or more of the vegetarians who have come to me because of their inability to conceive, have had their conception problems solved by reconstructing the damaged electrical circuitry of the reproductive system and dramatically increasing their protein intake, usually in the form of red meat.

The human body can only extract its life force, its vitality, from its nutritional intake. Children, as well as menstruating and breast feeding women, require high levels of protein intake to maintain their full vigor.

Protein is the main tissue builder of the body and is the basic substance of every cell, including muscles, bone, blood, skin, nails, hair and internal organs, hence the necessity for maintaining adequate levels of protein in our diet. Protein is essential for enzyme production, which enables electrical processes to take place. It is also important for the production of hormones which regulate and control bodily functions, including emotional stability.

I have found in my clinic that many young girls' emotional imbalances are dramatically helped by increasing the protein content of their diet, particularly red meat. Adequate levels of protein also assist in the production of antibodies which helps build the immune system.

We meet many typical vegetarians on our travels who are quiet spoken, listless, and totally lacking in vitality and passion. One woman in particular comes to mind. Her skin complexion was incredibly pale and she looked as if there was literally no meat on her bones. It was as if she were being eaten from the inside out and all her energy was depleted by the necessity of her body's survival without adequate nutritional backup. She was using up all her reserves and mining her body.

She typifies many young vegetarians who look just as unhealthy, if not more so, than overweight Burger King armchair sports addicts. Neither has a balanced understanding of nutrition.

This sadly is indicative of the long term vegetarians I have seen over the last fifteen years as part of my natural health practice. It was this startling reality that started me to question our entire nutritional understanding. People were coming to me at what should have been the prime of their lives, twenty to thirty years old, who had been strict vegetarians for ten or more years, and their bodies were literally falling apart.

At first this shocked me and upon questioning, a familiar pattern emerged. When they first became vegetarians some improvement in their health, vigor and vitality was noticed. Then, after five years or so, on a strict vegetarian diet, their vitality started to drop. By ten years, on a vegetarian diet, chronic malnourishment started to manifest in multiple areas of their physical body and entire systems were starting to shut down.

Some of the symptoms of vegetarianism that have become very easy for me to recognize are extreme paleness, suggesting a lack of amino acids and iron; lack of skin tone and deep sunken eyes, which signifies major mineral deficiencies; dark areas immediately under the eyes, signifying liver and kidney stress; and many times they show chronic low vitality that manifests as extremely low, to no libido in the males, period irregularity or none at all in the females, coupled with severe conception difficulties.

One of the most complained of symptoms is digestive disorders. If a client mentions digestive problems, my immediate response now is to ask if he or she is a vegetarian. In fact, I have become so good at recognizing malnourishment pertaining to vegetarians in the Western world, that my accuracy rate is running at about ninety nine percent in identifying this lifestyle choice, before the client gives me this information. Put plainly, I can pick 'em a mile off.

Let me add here that I also know vegetarians who understand explicitly the necessity for adequate levels of protein and are very conscientious with regard to their dietary intakes and supplementation. Those vegetarians who are informed and aware of their body's needs do not suffer from the disadvantages of a meat-free, protein-deficient diet.

I chuckle to myself when I recall a good friend telling me that she will not have a vegetarian lover because they do not have enough "chi" (energy). "They are all poor lovers... weak, low energy men" (her quote, not mine). This of course may or may not be true and I cannot personally vouch for the sexual "chi" of men, vegetarian or otherwise, due to inexperience. However, the story gets even funnier because my friend was a strict vego herself.

Another of the misconceptions in our current thinking is that humans have an intestinal tract that is too long for the quick passing through of animal protein. This concept that our digestive tract is too long is based on a comparison to the length of the digestive tract of dogs. The theory has been that dogs can ingest meat safely because of their extremely short digestive tract and because of our longer digestive tract, meat becomes putrid in our bowels.

If our digestive processes are working harmoniously with the necessary enzymes, gut bacteria, amino acids and all the other parameters operating correctly, it is impossible for any food to become putrid in our bowels.

Correct digestion is controlled rotting; putrid bowels are the result of uncontrolled rotting. The length of our digestive tract has nothing to do with it. Human beings have been ingesting animal protein since year dot. We evolved eating animal protein, and we are still here. Many of the old cultures who had extremely healthy and disease-free bodies ate large portions of animal protein.

Animals that have a longer digestive tract than ours, such as cows, require this because of the extreme difficulty in extracting nutrients from plant-based material (vegetation). The cow regurgitates the plant material for repeat grinding by the teeth (chewing the cud) in an attempt to break open the cellulose wall of the cell structure.

In excess of eighty percent of the cows internal energy gets used up in the process of digesting plant-based food. Only twenty percent of what the cow ingests is available for her life expression, the other eighty percent is used for digestion. On the other hand, the dog, with its extremely short digestive tract, has difficulty digesting vegetable matter but has a system perfectly capable of fermenting meat and extracting its nutrients.

The dogs input/usage ratio is far greater than that of a cow. A dog only uses twenty percent of its energy in the digestive process. Remember the life force availability in the Rock to Rot theory in Chapter Three.

Therefore, it is obvious that animal protein is a far more easily digested food, its nutrient extraction far more efficient than vegetation. Humans, with our medium length intestinal tract, have the obvious ability to extract all the nutrients from meat, and our digestive system is long enough to extract small percentages of the nutrients from grain-based foods and other vegetative matter.

I have always been amazed at how ill-informed some people are about the human intestinal tract's ability to digest animal protein because when we look at the records, one of the healthiest groups of people before White Man brought their sugar, were the Inuit Indians of Northern Canada.

Their diet for nine months of the year consisted solely of animal protein. They were known to have squeaky clean circulatory systems and be extremely well nourished in every way. The powerful bodies of the tribes of Africa, the amazing physique of the Pacific Island peoples (prior to civilization and our unnatural foods) were all developed with a predominance of animal protein as their diet. Degenerative diseases, including cancer, were unheard of. To suggest that the human intestinal tract cannot safely digest animal protein is to be a member of the flat earth society.

Animal protein gives us the highest return in energy availability, green vegetative matter is in the middle, and grains have the lowest return. Raw fresh fruit is right up there with animal proteins but only if ingested without other foods. Raw fruit does not require digestion. Mixing fruit with other food will start digestion and dramatically lower the body's ability to extract the energy from the fruit.

Another point that is often used as an excuse to suggest humans are not meant to ingest animal protein is that we do not have incisor teeth like the canines. The fact is, incisor teeth are not a requirement for the chewing of flesh. Our flat grinding teeth and jaw structure are more than capable of easily crushing and breaking open the cellular structure of flesh, as this is far easier than breaking open the cellular structure of cellulose cells of vegetative matter.

The only reason the canine species have incisor teeth is because, as the very word incisor means, to insert, the canine has to kill with its mouth. I have yet to see one with a bow and arrow or a gun. To pierce the thick hide and expose the jugular vein to make the kill, incisor teeth are necessary. The chewing of flesh is not a function of incisor teeth.

Thirty years ago, working farm dogs were fed a diet of one hundred percent meat and to have a sick dog, particularly one with cancer, was unheard of. Today, however, the average farmer often feeds his dogs hard food, which is commercially manufactured dog biscuits (cookies). These biscuits contain a large amount of vegetative matter, predominantly grains.

The digestive disorders and disease in the working dog is rampant and cancer is increasingly prevalent. This is also the case in a large percentage of domestic dogs and cats.

The length of our intestinal tract is just able to handle grains. It is not true that meat is difficult for humans to digest. It is, in fact, the most easily digestible food substance when combined correctly with an adequately functioning digestive system. Red meat gives us more nutrients, more amino acids, more iron, more protein for less work than any other known food source. The most complete and readily available source of the building blocks of life and vitality are contained in animal flesh.

From an electrical nutrition view point, animal flesh is the highest vibratory rate food and contains great amounts of life force, life force that becomes us. Vegetation is two steps down from us on the evolution ladder and therefore arguably, two steps lower in life force.

CHAPTER 6

GRAIN - AN ELECTRICAL DRAIN

For a number of years now, the big food fad in North America has been a high carbohydrate, grain-based diet. When I look down any busy American street, I see most people in various stages of obesity and degeneration. When I go into the malls, I see childhood obesity everywhere.

In the course of my year's work, I travel from Australasia to North America to Europe, and it is quite obvious that the obesity and disease levels in North America are by far the highest.

Once, I sat down in the food hall of a large mall and observed the busiest food stall. It was the bakery - a bakery of donuts, cinnamon buns and muffins, etc. Using the same observation technique, the most frequented aisles in the supermarket are those with the ready-made pasta and bread on the shelves. The ingestion of wheat in all its forms in North America far surpasses the nutritional requirements for carbohydrates.

When a farmer wants to fatten up a young cattle beast, he increases its grain ration. It responds instantly and gains weight directly to the ratio of the grain intake. But when he wants a milking cow to be lean, fit, able to conceive every year and produce gallons of milk per day (an energy requirement), he would lower the grain and increase the protein in her diet. An old farm saying is, "protein for production, grain for gain."

These basic nutritional facts have been known in agriculture for years, yet still do not seem to be understood by what we would term traditional nutritionists. The equation is simple:

If you want to slow your body down, make it heavy, not feel like moving and gain weight, then ingest a high-grain diet - eat lots of wheat products like bread, hamburger buns, donuts and pasta.

If you want to be full of vitality with lots of get up and go, with good muscle definition, i.e. be lean and fit, then have a high-protein diet.

From an energy perspective, digestion can use up to eighty percent of the body's internal energy. We know that grains have the highest energy requirement for digestion (grains take a lot of rotting), so eating a hearty muesli breakfast in the morning will give you exactly the opposite effect of what you thought you were going to achieve.

Rather than gaining lots of energy for movement or brain power, your body will want to shut down systems in order to supply the required energy for digestion.

Remember how you felt after your last big Thanksgiving/ Christmas dinner - all you wanted to do was sleep. This was because digestion has priority over all other body functions. **The fermenting of the food is an absolute priority**. Without fermentation taking place you would die, so the body shuts down all unnecessary functions. In extreme cases, like after a big dinner, it even shuts down the energy to stay awake. The body diverts all its energy to the digestive process. **You might "feel" sleepy, but the reality is that your body has enforced the shut down in a life-saving act.**

The hearty breakfast concept is, in fact, a carry over from an old English class one-up-man-ship. Back in the days of the landed gentry, the working classes had to work all day and as payment were given one of the hunted rabbits, pheasants or bag of grain to take home to the farm cottage, to be made into the main meal of the day for the family.

The Lords of the manor, on the other hand, did not have to work a day for their food and as a mark of their class, they had their main meal in the morning. The hearty breakfast originated as a class distinction and had nothing to do with good nutritional concepts.

If you desire to have lots of energy, to move, think and be active in the morning, then raw fresh fruit will supply you that energy. Fruit is more immediately available without the energy-hungry digestive process needed for grains.

Years ago when I was dairy farming milking five hundred cows, the normal routine was to come in from morning milking and eat the "hearty breakfast." What a breakfast: porridge with a half a cup of sugar and a cup of real cream on it, followed by bacon, eggs, hash browns and toast, all washed down with milk coffee (the new fancy city name for this farmers' coffee would be latte). Upon finishing this incredible feast, my body would shut down so quickly to ensure that digestion would have enough energy to function, I would fall asleep at the breakfast table.

Learning to understand how the body worked, my family and I were inspired to change our eating habits. Rising at 5 a.m. to milk the cows, I would take with me one banana and usually two other pieces of juicy fruit and work nonstop until lunch time and often beyond into mid-afternoon. My work output, my vitality and my waistline all improved dramatically. I have never gone back to a big breakfast since (unless I have a pig-out day and become a couch potato, just to remind myself how good it tastes and how bad it feels…I'm still human!).

Looking at wheat, from an electrical nutrition perspective, it is clear that the vibratory rate of wheat is such that its ability to nourish the human body is relatively low. If we ingest wheat in an unground form, like in whole-grain breads, that grain of wheat will pass through our intestinal tract totally unfermented, undigested and completely intact.

Or, if you threw some wheat out on the ground and waited for it to decompose, you would be waiting a long time. Sure, things get a hurry-up in the fermentation tank called our stomach, but even then that whole grain of wheat is hardly broken down before it gets eliminated.

That is why we have learnt from the old cultures to grind our grains before we ingest them. Only some birds can take in whole grain and get nourishment from it. But then again, our friendly common hen carries with it its own grinding device called a crop. Within that crop there are stones, bits of glass, broken crockery if its available, and any other very hard matter that the hen can find. She regurgitates the whole grain into this crop and flexing her muscles, grinds it.

A hen can eat almost anything and digest it. In fact, their digestive process is far more efficient than ours and even with that efficiency the hen still has to grind that grain to oblivion. Humans think they are being so healthy by ingesting whole grains! Whole grains are useless to us from a nutritional point of view. But they do make good fiber, which our body will use in an attempt to scour the walls of our colon clean. Then again, if we did not have a half an inch of gunk around the inside wall of our colon, we would not need this scouring effect.

So what do crushed grains, as in flour, do for us? One of the things ingesting wheat does is to set up a high probability of joint degeneration. Once again, this has been known to agricultural science for in excess of fifty years. In the dairy industry, an excess of crushed grain in the feed stock would give cows hotfoot, i.e. extremely tender and swollen leg joints. In horses, too much grain in their diet can lead to a symptom called foundering.

In human beings, wheat or grain toxicity takes a little longer to manifest because our bodies are so amazingly evolved that they convert any excess carbohydrate into cellulite (fat) and put it away for the next famine. And we all know where our bodies put it!

After a number of years of attempting to deal with this excess grain intake, the electrical circuitry starts to fail and we feel this in the joints. If you want to guarantee joint degeneration problems from middle age on, eat a lot of grain-based foods.

In my clinical experience, I have seen arthritic symptoms, tender, swollen and painful joints, all successfully alleviated when clients have taken all grain and sugar from their diet. This is followed by increasing their protein intake and adding an electrically formulated herbal bowel cleanse and enzymes into their nutritional program (more about this later).

In my opinion, the over-consumption of grain in North America is largely responsible for the chronic obesity, adult onset diabetes, lethargy and joint degeneration that is so prevalent. When we combine this high-grain intake with sugar, we produce in our body a substance that is electrically devastating and that dramatically slows down cell function.

Do not forget when flour is mixed with water it makes glue (when we were kids we made the most awesome kites out of brown paper and we glued them all together with flour and water glue). Flour and sugar will clog up and destroy the human body quicker than any other food combination, including the meat and potato scenario.

It is frightening that a large percentage of juveniles in North America are fed such a diet. Their daily intake normally consists of pop, donuts, muffins, burgers, noodles, pasta, hot-dog buns and various other grain and sugar based foods.

This is the perfect recipe for obesity, endocrine system malfunction, emotional instability and often leads to reproductive system problems with the young women - painful and difficult periods being one of the first symptoms. Skin eruptions, acne, chronic irritability, concentration deficits and general learning difficulties are all early manifestations of serious grain and sugar toxicity.

In our older population, as well as the obvious obesity symptom, lethargy, libido problems, conception problems, menopausal difficulties later in life, prostrate symptoms in men and of course the big one, joint degeneration and arthritis are all long term symptoms of grain toxicity and excess sugar.

One of the most prevalent grain toxicity disorders, which very few people realize is 100% induced by excess grain intake, is the "disease" commonly referred to as adult onset diabetes. This so-called "disease," in my clinical experience, often has more than a 95% reversal when the clients take all of the grain out of their diet for a period of at least six months. However, most people never go back onto grain after that time because they realize how devastating it was to their body and how yucky and heavy they feel when they do eat it. By grain obviously we mean all bread, pasta, donuts, pizza, cereals, cookies, etc. anything that has been made from any grain, particularly wheat being the worst offender.

Nature in her wisdom wrapped up the seed-head in a fibrous tissue and designed it so that it was un-rottable. A seed-head can get blown away in the wind, washed away in the flood, sit under six feet of snow, and it does not rot. The only way nature has designed grain to give its life force, is through the process of germination and the resulting sprout, which is then a complex protein, or the "flesh" of the plant, which is now available to the animals, digestive tract. Our body, and in particular our digestive tract, has an almost total inability to ferment a seed-head whether it is whole or ground up. Nature designed the seed-head to store the life-giving energy and when we try to eat grain, the innate frequency of the seed-head can only go into storage, ie. lay down cellulite. That is why in agriculture, to fatten up the hog on the farm we feed it grain. Grain is the hardest thing to ferment, takes the most energy, and we get little or nothing from it, except large thighs, butts and bellies.

If we as a society are going to take stock of our rapidly rising health problems, we had better start to understand some basic fundamentals about electrical nutrition. Our bodies have a small requirement for carbohydrate and many people choose to use rice, but when I look at the nutritional content of rice it always amazes me that anybody would willingly eat rice when in most of the western world we have an abundance of readily-available potatoes.

From an electrically available nutritional point of view, the humble spud should be our carbohydrate of choice. Because of its interaction with our body's electrical matrix, **it cannot cause obesity**, does not clog the lymphatic system (if not combined with protein) and supplies more amino acids and various other building blocks of life than any of the grains. The potato is one of the least altered foods we eat. It is as nature designed it and that is why it is electrically available to us. Its electrical matrix has a seamless interface with ours. Potatoes are a great food for maintaining blood/sugar levels.

Grains, and in particular wheat, have to be ground to be of any use to us. Stripped, with many of its components separated from its original form, its electrical matrix is no longer the way nature made it, so its energy availability, from an electrical nutrition standpoint, is severely depleted.

From an electrical nutrition understanding, modern grains could well be considered toxic.

However, sweet corn, from an electrical nutrition view point, would be the least damaging grain, with all other grains in between.

The modern farming practice, with its chemical fertilizers, artificial breeding of grain cultivars and soil nutrient deficiencies, produces wheat that has very little relationship to the wheat plant of even twenty years ago. Of all the crops grown, wheat is one of the most chemically sprayed crops there is.

The lowering of our grain quality is largely unknown by the general populace. Due to the poor quality of our grains, the electrical matrix is exceedingly different from what it was. Modern grains are responsible for the laying down of cellulite (fat) more than any other food. The cellulite then holds toxins from other chemically-laced foods, and in fact becomes the body's very convenient toxic waste dump. The choice is yours.

CHAPTER 7

THE ELECTRICAL MATRIX OF FOOD

Looking at the concepts of what is good food and what is not, once again we have to move away from the old paradigm of conventional nutritional thinking.

From a nutritional point of view, everything we do to our food changes its subtle electrical reality, its electrical matrix, and how it interfaces with our body.

Using the example of melting some tin and melting some lead and then mixing the two molten materials together and allowing them to solidify (cool down, lower their frequency), what results is very different than the two components we started with.

The behavior, or physical properties, of our new alloy, called solder, is exceedingly different from either of, or the sum total of, the two components. In other words, everything about it now is different. The most startling physical difference is solder's melting point, which is now way below tin or lead. What has actually changed is its electrical matrix, its electrical construct, the way the neutrons and protons and electrons arrange themselves.

Also, if we look at ice, water and humidity, we can see that as we change the electrical matrix of an H_2O molecule, the resulting physicality and its interface with everything around it changes. If you do not think ice has a different physicality to water, I am sure that if he was alive, the captain of the Titanic would give you a good argument.

We can breathe single H_2O molecules as in humidity, but we cannot see it. Water, however as three and four H_2O ($3H_2O$ or $4H_2O$) molecules would kill us if we tried to breath it, yet we cannot survive without drinking it. And ice will break our bones if we try diving in it, and I have never seen a fish swim in ice.

I hope these examples help you understand that as soon as we change the electrical matrix of anything, we change the way it then interfaces with everything else. In other words, change the matrix of protons and electrons, their electrical construct, and everything about them changes - their physicality, appearance, frequency… everything.

Likewise, everything we do to our food: the way we fertilize it, spray it, drench it, heat it, wash it, dry it, mix it, take bits out of it, put bits into it, irradiate it, preserve it, color it, flavor it, freeze it etc., changes its electrical matrix.

What we store food in and every human contact the food has affects its electrical make-up. From the farmer who touched the seed or the animal, to the check-out person at the supermarket, all have infused a frequency of energy into that food. Then of course, the person who is preparing the food for our ingestion has a profound effect on its frequency (the movie "Like Water for Chocolate" is a good demonstration of this).

Nature, which we are a part of, designed an electrical matrix between the food chain and ourselves that allowed the energy that is the nutritional frequencies to be seamlessly available to us. Our so-called technology, particularly in the last thirty years, has literally changed the electrical matrix of every piece of food we buy from the supermarket.

Hopefully, it is becoming glaringly obvious we are unconsciously poisoning ourselves. Due to our one-sided education, we have not taken into consideration the electrical understanding of what food is and what it does. I hope to show you that you can do something about making your food electrically available again.

Two hundred years ago, before the advent of modern agriculture, everything we planted, grew and ate contained the electrical matrix nature had developed over tens of thousands of years. All our medicine came from the knowledge of herbs that had been built up since time began.

There was hardly any evidence of the diseases and problems we live with today, such as cancer, fibromyalgia, cystic fibrosos, PMS, AIDS, multiple sclerosis, autism, congenital adrenal hyperplasia, Alzheimers, etc.

The water we were drinking back then was completely free of the toxic loading of our modern industrial age. It certainly did not have the toxic substances man has produced that have absolutely no electrical synergy with the body, such as chlorine, arsenic, acetone, chloride, carbon tetrachloride, as well as mercury, lead, aluminum, fluoride, and petro chemical distillates.

When we look at every aspect of our present environment, we have to come to the conclusion that we have changed everything we interface with.

Soil developed as a result of tens of thousands of years of microbacteria converting rocks and vegetable matter into live topsoil. When the pioneer farmers first started to farm the Midwest plains in the U.S. there was in excess of six feet of top soil. Today there is *very* much less. Our entire natural base for food production no longer exists.

There is hardly one vegetable that is commercially grown in North America that is the same cultivar, that has the same genetic makeup, or contains the same electrical matrix that nourished our great grandparents. What was in the soil two hundred years ago is now long gone. Our food is only capable of being as healthy as the soil.

Everything above the ground is a reflection of what is going on below the ground. In our great grandmothers' day, every time we ate a fruit or vegetable we got nature's bountiful basket that not only contained the carrot we may have been eating but also contained within that carrot, enzymes and micro bacteria that were living in the soil.

As a result of ingesting all of these components, our stomach got repopulated with natural bacteria and flora with every mouthful. The alive, healthy soil was transferred to us in most of the food we ate. Today, a large proportion of the micro bacteria and enzymes that populated the soil two hundred years ago do not exist. From an electrical nutrition understanding, this is a disaster.

Our bodies have evolved over millions of years on earth, so any change is an extremely slow process. This evolution took place in an environment of total electrical compatibility with the rest of nature, which included our food. It is not difficult to understand that by changing the electrical matrix of the soil and our food in a dramatically short period of time, our bodies are now virtually incapable of being in electrical harmony with the food.

What we perceive as nutrition is, in fact, an illusion. Wonderful looking fruits and vegetables are, in fact, not what they seem. The compatibility between the electrical matrix of the food and the electrical matrix of our bodies is out of harmony. The electrical synergy between our food and us has to be correct, otherwise food becomes a poison. This is pure electrical science. The long-term ingestion of low level poisons leads to electrical disharmony which we label as diseases.

In an attempt to keep our soil productive, the modern farmer has no option other than to use chemical compounds and fertilizers. The more enlightened ones also test their soil for mineral balance and replace the necessary minerals if deficiencies occur. However, one of the big distinctions between raising crops and animals is that it is very easy to have exceedingly good-looking and high-yielding crops using only the NPK (nitrogen, phosphate and potassium) formula.

With this formula, the resulting crops may well have chronic mineral deficiencies, but without complex analysis this is not apparent. Very rarely does any cereal manufacturer, baker, or food manufacturer pay the farmer on the mineral or micronutrient content of the crop. Normally, the farmer gets paid by the ton and can survive economically only by producing tonnages. The NPK model will produce lots of tonnage.

On the other hand, animals will very quickly show symptoms of mineral and micronutrient deficiencies. Therefore, the farmer who raises animals has to be much more aware of micronutrient and other nutritional requirements.

Mineral and vitamin supplementation has been part of the agricultural scene for many years. In fact, there would not be a cattle farmer out there who did not know the importance of balanced nutrition. At times minerals and micronutrients will be added to the feed mix because if there are a few thousand head of cattle on a feed lot and the feed ration had a vitamin or mineral deficiency in it, the farmer, very quickly, would be facing a multi-million dollar catastrophe in the form of very sick and dying animals. So, purely from a balanced nutritional sense, the animal production system is giving us a healthier, more balanced option.

If our agricultural production has understood the need for mineral supplementation for many years, why has our so-called medical system denied, and in fact, actively campaigned against the fortification of our diet in the form of mineral, herbal and vitamin supplementation?

It was back in 1936 that the United States government was informed of soil nutrient problems, and I quote from U.S. Senate Document No 264.

"The alarming fact is that foods (fruits, vegetables and grains) now being raised on millions of acres of land that no longer contains enough of certain minerals, are starving us - no matter how much we eat. No man of today can eat enough fruits and vegetables to supply his system with the minerals he requires for perfect health because his stomach isn't big enough to hold them."

"The truth is that our foods vary enormously in value, and some of them aren't worth eating as food... Our physical well-being is more directly dependent upon the minerals we take into our system than upon calories or vitamins or upon the precise proportions of starch, protein or carbohydrates we consume."

AND THAT WAS BACK IN 1936.

It often intrigued me that a can of a popular brand of cat food, lists forty-two vitamin and mineral additives that were said to be essential for the healthy life of our feline friend. Yet two aisles away in the same supermarket, the cans of baby food contained only eight of the same nutritional supplements. Why is it that veterinary science which was responsible for formulating the cat food saw the importance of the micronutrients and minerals while our human nutritionists, including doctors, do not see the same importance for our children? The contents of both cans came from the same agricultural base, from the same nutrient-deficient soil.

Agricultural science is motivated for the reason of preventing the manifestation of disease in the farm animals for its economic survival. **On the other hand, the economic survival of the human medical system depends on illness** (there would be no need for doctors and drugs if there were no illness). Face it, if all human diseases stopped tomorrow there would be one tremendous hiccup in the world's financial system.

On the other hand, if the same amount of disease that exists in humans was allowed to manifest in the farming scene, the disruption to our food supply would result in mass starvation. The two health care systems operate from opposite ends of the spectrum.

Understanding our food production system, the depletion of our soils, the mineral deficiencies in grain and vegetable production, the lack of adequate animal protein in our diet, and our obsession with grain/sugar-based products such as donuts, pasta, hot-dogs, burgers and pop, it is easy to see the reason for our chronic disease manifestation.

It is impossible for our bodies to function electrically in perfect harmony with the imbalanced electrical matrix that is our modern diet.

To correct this electrical and dietary disharmony, we need the supplementation of electrically-available minerals, herbs, enzymes and natural bacterias.

If it is good enough for veterinary science to supplement cat food to make it nutritionally correct, it is about time we accepted this for ourselves and our children.

The human dietary supplementation intake has enjoyed an exponential growth in the last ten years, despite the originally negative rumblings from the pharmaceutical industry that supplements were not necessary. The same pharmaceutical industry now predominantly manufactures the raw material, for the biggest percentage of supplements. The worldwide swing to nutritional supplementation was obviously a market that the pharmaceutical companies could not ignore.

However these pharmaceutical companies manufacture the nutritional supplements (which are predominantly sold in Drugstores and Health Food stores) from the basis of traditional chemical medicine, by following the old paradigm of particle physics, not from an electrical perspective. If our traditional scientific and pharmaceutical industry refuses to accept the leading-edge research into the electrical universe, there is no possibility that the nutritional supplements being produced can be electrically available to the body.

How is it possible for our bodies to maintain full and vigorous health, i.e. full electrical function, if the soil our food is grown in has been distorted, if the food we eat is anaemic and the supplementation we take to try and correct the problems is manufactured with the same thinking, the same "science" that has caused all the problems in the first place?

Supplementation up until now has not worked very well. We are still sick and disease-ridden. We obviously need a new source of nutritional supplements that are electrically available to the body. Supplements must be formulated with the understanding of the whole electrical process.

This is where a small section of scientists is going. The research into the electrical compatibility of different herbs and minerals and their correct electrical interface with the cells in our bodies is at the top end of nutritional science. There are formulators who have used electrical compatibility knowledge and formulated some of the world's most advanced electrically-available natural nutritional supplements. (Refer to Appendix)

We now have health-giving products that act the way nature and our bodies work - electrically. These products and their ability to interface with our bodies, to detox and reverse the degeneration that we call disease, are light years ahead of anything we ever had previously. We are talking about a completely different set of rules, electrical rules, that until now we did not know existed.

Prior to this electrically available knowledge, the industry standard for the absorbability of nutritional supplements had been around ten percent. That is why many doctors and others have said taking supplements has been a waste of time. It is only now - in the last two to four years - that electrically formulated products, with an availability to the cells that at times exceeds ninety percent, have been available through mail-order health clubs and other high-end retail health professionals.

Ten years ago we had no knowledge of the importance of electrical availability in anything, let alone our food or supplementation. Quantum physics is working towards this realization, the realization that everything interfaces with everything else on an energy level. For doctors and nutritionists to have closed minds regarding electrical availability and the wholesale destruction to the body caused by the electrical matrix being changed, is to be ignorant of leading scientific knowledge.

It is sad but true that change is slow to take hold. This is especially true in the health and medical fields. It is probably even more true when some new knowledge comes along that requires a complete one hundred and eighty degree turn and in the process we have to get our logic around a completely different set of parameters.

One such change that was slow to take hold occurred in the middle of the 19th century, and I quote from, "Reclaiming Our Health" by John Robbind, 1996,

Ignaz Semmelweis, a young obstetrician who delivered babies in a famous Viennese hospital noticed women coming to give birth were sent to one of the hospital's two sections - the First Clinic, where obstetricians prevailed and medical students received training, or the Second Clinic, staffed entirely by midwives. Noticing that woman were literally begging to be admitted to the Second Clinic, Semmelweis began to look carefully at the autopsy records from the two sections. What he discovered was that the death rate from puerperal (childbed) fever for woman in the "doctor's" wards was more that four times higher than for woman under the midwives' jurisdiction.

Semmelweis, like other doctors of his time, had no idea that (some) germs could cause disease. This was some twenty years before Joseph Lister would advance the use of antiseptics in surgery. But, in a moment of inspiration, he decreed that the medical students handling deliveries on his ward should wash their hands in a chlorine solution after dissecting corpses, and after each examination of a woman in the ward.

The results were outstanding. Before the hand washing, one out of every eight woman giving birth in the First Clinic had died of puerperal fever. But now the death rate dropped almost immediately to less than 1 in 100.

What do you think the reaction was when Semmelweis published the records of this spectacular success? Was he heralded and applauded, and his ideas immediately put into practice in all obstetrical clinics?

Not quite; Orthodox obstetricians virtually declared war on the poor man, battering and insulting him at every opportunity. He was hounded from Vienna and eventually driven insane by the relentless attacks. He died without ever knowing that his views would eventually triumph, and thanks to his discoveries, (or was it the midwives that he learned it from) puerperal fever would nearly disappear.

Why were such spectacular results dismissed by the medical establishment of the day? (Was it that) members of the medical establishment were at that time implacably resistant to any insinuation that their own practices were harming (women).

Sadly, sometimes I have to ask, "So what has changed?"

I hope the concept of electrical nutrition is accepted more readily. When we embrace the electrical universe, we have to come to terms with the reality of everything being an electrical construct, carrying within itself an electrical matrix and interfacing with everything on an electrical or energy level. To change any component of the matrix is to effect change and behavior to the whole.

This concept totally displaces the particle physics mindset and reassigns chemistry to kindergarten logic. We live in an electrical universe, we are electrical, and everything we interface with is electrical. **Everything is an electrical action,** not a chemical reaction. This fundamental concept is the change of consciousness we have all been searching for. This can and will lead us to enlightenment.

I am now going to share with you two reports that came my way that graphically demonstrate the unbelievable chaos and "integrity fraud" that the food manufacturing, pharmaceutical companies and government departments all perpetrate. I and others have mentioned many times over the years the electrical disaster that is sugar, but sadly its common replacement that comes under the trade names of NutraSweet, Equal and Spoonful and others that contain Aspartame are possibly even more potent poisons. I will leave you to decide after reading these two reports (these reports are unaltered and reprinted as they came to me, thank you to those involved).

Report one.

Alzheimers is not only triggered by aluminum although it is one reason for the disease. Dr. H.J. Roberts has done 30 years of research on Alzheimers and has just published a book on it called DEFENSE AGAINST ALZHEIMER DISEASE (1-800-814-9800). It has been nominated for a Pulitzer and is a very knowledgeable and incredible book written with great dignity, understanding and compassion. Dr. Roberts was here in Atlanta giving a seminar and went into some things that can trigger Alzheimers (such as zinc). When aspartame (marketed as NutraSweet, Equal, Spoonful, etc.), was approved, Dr. Roberts noticed a big difference in his diabetic and multiple sclerosis patients. (Dr. Roberts is a diabetic specialist.) They showed memory loss, confusion, and serious vision problems. He goes into this in his book. Alzheimers is a 20th century disease and is now the fourth leading cause of death in adults in the U.S. (4 million victims).

Dr. Roberts says that the two amino acids in aspartame are neurotoxic without the other amino acids in protein (phenylalanine and aspartic acid). They go past the blood brain barrier and deteriorate the neurons of the brain. This is the cause of Alzheimers. Dr. Roberts says, in his opinion, NutraSweet is escalating Alzheimers. There are 250,000 new cases each year and 100,000 deaths. Fifty percent of all patients in nursing homes are Alzheimers patients (including mature baby boomers). A couple of days ago a nursing assistant told me she was just shocked that now 30 year old women are being admitted with Alzheimers! After all, NutraSweet comes in its own aluminum can! Aspartame is nothing but a chemical poison. It has methyl ester in it that becomes methanol (wood alcohol), and in the body it converts to formaldehyde and formic acid (ant sting poison) and causes metabolic acidosis!

It is disastrous for a diabetic patient even though it is recommended by the American Diabetic Association, but that's because they are funded by Monsanto. Dr. Roberts has been a member for almost forty years and gave them an abstract of diabetic aspartame reactors but they refused to publish it. It was published in Clinical Research (Vol. 36, No. 3, 1988, 489A). I suspect they can't warn the diabetics this is a poison and at the same time, continue to take money from its manufacturer, Monsanto. You can be sure around October 1, the NutraSweet Company (Monsanto) will sponsor walk-a-thons for the ADA and distribute Equal shirts. One big problem is that diabetic patients can have diabetic retinopathy.

Many physicians don't realize when they [diabetics] are consuming aspartame what is really happening is that the patients are going blind. The methanol (wood alcohol), that blinded and killed skid row drunks during prohibition, converts to formaldehyde in the retina of the eye. That's why so many bleed and have retinal detachments. It's very tragic.

Even Dr. Russell Blaylock, neurosurgeon, who wrote EXCITOTOXINS: THE TASTE THAT KILLS, says that the ingredients in NutraSweet literally stimulate the neurons of the brain to death causing damage of varying degrees. This is written on the back of his book. He also says that aspartame can even trigger diabetes. It is no wonder that there are so many diabetics in this country.

The FDA in August 1995 listed the following symptoms from aspartame: Headaches, dizziness or balance problems, change in mood quality or level, vomiting and nausea, abdominal pain and cramps, change in vision, diarrhea, seizures and convulsions, memory loss, fatigue, weakness, rash, sleep problems, hives, change in heart rate, itching, change in sensation (numbness, tingling), grand mal seizures, local swelling, change in activity level, difficulty breathing, oral sensory changes, change in menstrual pattern, other localized pain and tenderness, other urogenital problems, body temperature changes, swallowing difficulty, other metabolic problems, joint and bone pain, speech impairment, miscellaneous gastrointestinal problems, chest pain, other musculo-skeletal problems, fainting, sore throat, other cardiovascular problems, change in taste, difficulty with urination, other respiratory problems, edema, change in hearing, change in perspiration pattern, eye irritation, unspecified muscle tremors, petit mal, change in body weight, change in thirst or water intake, unconsciousness and coma, wheezing, constipation, other extremity pain, problems with bleeding, unsteady gait, coughing, blood glucose disorders, blood pressure changes, changes in skin and nail coloration, change in hair or nails, excessive phlegm production, sinus problems, simple partial seizures, hallucinations, any lumps present, dysmenorrehea, dental problems, change in smell, DEATH, other blood and lymphatic problems, eczema, complex partial seizures, swollen lymph nodes, hematuria, shortness of breath, difficulties with pregnancy, developmental retardation in children, change in breast size or tenderness, change in sexual function, shock, conjunctivitis, dilating eyes.

If you saw these many adverse reactions in the Physicians Desk Reference (PDR) of drugs, would you consider taking it?

Actually, it is a drug and was discovered by a Seattle chemist testing a peptic ulcer drug. Notice how they throw DEATH in the middle of those symptoms. Nice little sweetener! Barbara Mullarkey, a journalist in Oak Park, Illinois, has written about aspartame since it was approved and has written about those symptoms before. One article was titled: DEATH: THE ULTIMATE SYMPTOM!

Keep in mind when there were congressional hearings in Washington, aspartame was only in a few hundred products, but now the patent has expired and it is in 5000 products! You've got this drug in your coffee, in your soda, ice cream, gum, over the counter drugs, and prescription medications, and even in baked goods. You cannot heat aspartame because it becomes a witches brew of breakdown products, but the FDA forgot they said not to heat it and approved it in baked goods in 1993.

Do you wonder why it is triggering all these neurological diseases? Anything that changes the brain chemistry is disastrous! You should see what it does to a Parkinson's patient because it changes the dopamine level.

Whoever said you cannot trust the FDA is right. This is the greatest atrocity the FDA ever committed in the history of this country. There was so much opposition to the approval of this drug that the DA set up a Board of Inquiry. They said not to approve aspartame because it caused brain tumors and grand mal seizures in lab animals just for starters! Yet, Dr. Arthur Hull Hayes, head of the FDA, overruled his own Board of Inquiry . . . And then conveniently went to work for Searles' Public Relations firm and refused to talk to the press for ten years. Monsanto bought Searle in 1985!

This product is causing an epidemic of chronic fatigue syndrome (methanol breaks down the immune system), systemic lupus and fibromyalgia. People are constantly being diagnosed with multiple sclerosis, when in reality they have methanol toxicity from aspartame, which mimics MS! We get the people off aspartame and usually within a couple of months the MS symptoms disappear - if we get to them in time! If any of you are using aspartame and are having vision problems, headaches, slurring of words, numbness, cramps, and shooting pains in your legs, vertigo, dizziness, tinnitus, joint pain, insomnia, etc., you could be suffering from methanol toxicity. Be assured it does kill!

Richard Wilson wrote in an Atlanta Newspaper in April, 1994:

"Aspartame killed my wife. No words can express the agony and horror sweet Joyce endured. The poison destroyed her brain, ravaged all her organs, and blinded her. She died at age 46 in 1996. . . . The makers of this poison considered her death an acceptable cost of business. I'm a man without a wife because the NutraSweet Company is a business without a conscience."

We are MISSION POSSIBLE, a volunteer force in 50 states, distributing a warning flyer worldwide on aspartame. If you would like one to distribute, just e-mail me for instructions. We also have other posts of interest and reports, and the history of aspartame. We ask all people on NutraSweet to take the 'no aspartame test' and then send us your case histories to help others. We also have available some of the case histories we've already taken off the net. It is lengthy but available to anyone who wants it. Joyce Wilson had the symptoms of MS which was the methanol toxicity, and when she died she was just like an Alzheimers victim with no memory! But until she could no longer remember, she tried to warn the world and testified before Congress. Like I said, Monsanto has deep pockets, her pleas fell on deaf ears. Even the late Dr. Adrian Goss, FDA toxicologist, told Congress that aspartame violated the Delaney Amendment because beyond a shadow of a doubt it caused cancer in lab animals.

His last words will never be forgotten: "If the FDA violates its own laws who is left to protect the people?" We have no protector so we must warn each other.

Patricia Craine is another victim of NutraSweet. Her death was reported on CBN. It was mentioned that her autopsy, a medically documented case like that of Joyce Wilson, was identical to that of Christina Onassis, a Diet Coke addict! It's not worth it folks. These people are living a nightmare and many times the physicians don't recognize the symptoms because they don't associate them with aspartame. They've been told by the organizations that sold out to Monsanto funding, that it is safe.

Mission Possible is dedicated to the proposition that we won't be satisfied until death and disability are no longer considered an acceptable cost of business.

Report Two:
"Aspartame - The Silent Killer."

I have spent several days lecturing at the WORLD ENVIRONMENTAL CONFERENCE on "ASPARTAME marketed as 'NutraSweet,' 'Equal' and 'Spoonful.'" In the keynote address by the EPA, they announced that there was an epidemic of multiple sclerosis and systemic lupus, and they did not understand what toxin was causing this to be rampant across the United States. I explained that I was there to lecture on exactly that subject.

When the temperature of Aspartame exceeds 86 degrees F, the wood alcohol in Aspartame coverts to formaldehyde and then to formic acid, which in turn causes metabolic acidosis. (Formic acid is the poison found in the sting of fire ants.) The methanol toxicity mimics multiple sclerosis; thus people were being diagnosed with having multiple sclerosis in error.

The multiple sclerosis is not a death sentence, where methanol toxicity is. In the case of systemic lupus, we are finding it has become almost as rampant as multiple sclerosis, especially [among] Diet Coke and Diet Pepsi drinkers. Also, with methanol toxicity, the victims usually drink three to four 12 oz. cans of them per day, some even more. In the cases of systemic lupus, which is triggered by Aspartame, the victim usually does not know that the Aspartame is the culprit. The victim continues its use, aggravating the lupus to such a degree that sometimes it becomes life threatening. When we get people off the Aspartame, those with systemic lupus usually become asymptomatic. Unfortunately, we can not reverse this disease.

On the other hand, in the case of those diagnosed with Multiple Sclerosis, (when in reality, the disease is methanol toxicity), most of the symptoms disappear. We have seen cases where their vision has returned and even their hearing has returned. This also applies to cases of tinnitus. During a lecture I said "If you are using Aspartame (NutraSweet, Equal, Spoonful, etc.) and you suffer from fibromyalgia symptoms, spasms, shooting pains, numbness in your legs, cramps, vertigo, dizziness, headaches, tinnitus, joint pain, depression, anxiety attacks, slurred speech, blurred vision, or memory loss - you probably have Aspartame Disease!"

People were jumping up during the lecture saying, "I've got this, is it reversible?" It is rampant. Some of the speakers at my lecture even were suffering from these symptoms. In one lecture attended by the Ambassador of Uganda, he told us that their sugar industry is adding Aspartame! He continued by saying that one of the industry leader's sons could no longer walk - due in part by product usage!

We have a serious problem. Even a stranger came up to Dr. Espisto (one of my speakers) and myself and said, 'Could you tell me why so many people seem to be coming down with MS?' During a visit to a hospice, a nurse said that six of her friends, who were heavy Diet Coke addicts, had all been diagnosed with MS. This is beyond coincidence.

Here is the problem. There were Congressional Hearings when Aspartame was included in 100 different products. Since this initial hearing, there have been two subsequent hearings, but to no avail. Nothing has been done. The drug and chemical lobbies have very deep pockets. Now there are over 5,000 products containing this chemical, and the PATENT HAS EXPIRED!!!!!

Aspartame can be found in:
  * *Instant breakfasts, gelatin desserts, soft drinks and pop*
  * *Breath mints, juice beverages, tabletop sweeteners*
  * *Cereals, laxatives, tea beverages*
  * *Sugar-free chewing gum, multivitamins, instant coffees and teas*
  * *Cocoa mixes, milk drinks, topping mixes*
  * *Coffee beverages, pharmaceuticals & health supplements, wine coolers, frozen desserts, shake mixes, yogurt etc.*

At the time of this first hearing, people were going blind. The methanol in the Aspartame converts to formaldehyde in the retina of the eye. Formaldehyde is grouped in the same class of drugs as cyanide and arsenic - DEADLY POISONS!!! Unfortunately, it just takes longer to quietly kill, but it is killing people and causing all kinds of neurological problems. Aspartame changes the brain's chemistry. It is the reason for severe seizures. This drug changes the dopamine level in the brain. Imagine what this drug does to patients suffering from Parkinson's Disease. This drug also causes birth defects.

There is absolutely no reason to take this product. It is NOT A DIET PRODUCT!!! The Congressional record said, "It makes you crave carbohydrates and [they] will make you FAT." Dr. Roberts stated that when he got patients off Aspartame, their average weight loss was 19 pounds per person. The formaldehyde stores in the fat cells, particularly in the hips and thighs.

Aspartame is especially deadly for diabetics. All physicians know what wood alcohol will do to a diabetic. We find that physicians believe that they have patients with retinopathy, when in fact, it is caused by the Aspartame. The Aspartame keeps the blood sugar level out of control, causing many patients to go into coma. Unfortunately, many have died.

People were telling us at the Conference of the American College of Physicians that they had relatives that switched from saccharin to an Aspartame product and how that relative had eventually gone into a coma. Their physicians could not get the blood sugar levels under control. Thus the patients suffered acute memory loss and eventually coma and death.

Memory loss is due to the fact that aspartic acid and phenylalanine are neurotoxic without the other amino acids found in protein. Thus is goes past the blood brain barrier and deteriorates the neurons of the brain. Dr. Russell Blaylock, neurosurgeon, said, "The ingredients stimulate the neurons of the brain to death, causing brain damage of varying degrees." Dr. Blaylock has written a book entitled "EXCITOTOXINS: THE TASTE THAT KILLS" (Health Press 1-800-643-2665).

Dr. H.L. Roberts, diabetic specialist and world expert on aspartame poisoning, has also written a book entitled "DEFENSE AGAINST ALZHEIMER'S DISEASE" (1-800-814-9800). Dr. Roberts tells how aspartame poisoning is escalating Alzheimers disease and indeed it is. As the hospice nurse told me, women are being admitted at 30 years of age with Alzheimers Disease. Dr. Blaycock and Dr. Roberts will be writing a position paper with some case histories and will post it on the Internet. According to the Conference of the American College of Physicians, "We are talking about a plague of neurological diseases caused by this deadly poison."

Dr. Roberts realized what was happening when aspartame was first marketed. He said, "many diabetic patients presented memory loss, confusion, and severe vision loss."

At the Conference of the American College of Physicians, doctors admitted that they did not know. They had wondered why seizures were rampant (the phenylalanine in aspartame breaks down the seizure threshold and depletes serotonin, which causes manic depression, panic attacks, rage and violence). Just before the Conference, I received a fax from Norway, asking for a possible antidote for this poison because they are experiencing so many problems in their country.

This "poison" is now available in 90-plus countries worldwide. Fortunately, we had speakers and ambassadors at the Conference from different nations who have pledged their help. We ask that you help too.

Print this article out and warn everyone you know. Take anything that contains aspartame back to the store. Take the "NO ASPARTAME TEST" and send us your case history. I assure you that MONSANTO, the creator of aspartame, knows how deadly it is. They fund the American Diabetes Association, American Dietetic Association Congress, and the Conference of the American College of Physicians.

The New York Times, on November 15, 1996, ran an article on how the American Dietetic Association takes money from the food industry to endorse their products. Therefore, they can not criticize any additives or tell about their link to MONSANTO. How bad is this?

We told a mother who had a child on NutraSweet to get off the product. The child was having grand mal seizures every day. The mother called her physician, who called the ADA, who told the doctor not to take the child off the NutraSweet. We are still trying to convince the mother that the aspartame is causing the seizures. Every time we get someone off aspartame, the seizures stop. If the baby dies, you know whose fault it is, and what we are up against.

There are 92 documented symptoms of aspartame, from coma to death. The majority of them are all neurological, because the aspartame destroys the nervous system.

Aspartame disease is partially the cause to what is behind some of the mystery of the Dessert Storm health problems. The burning tongue and other problems discussed in over 60 cases can be directly related to the consumption of an aspartame product. Several thousand pallets of diet drinks were shipped to the Dessert Storm troops. (Remember heat can liberate the methanol from the aspartame at 86 degrees F.) Diet drinks sat in the 120 degree F. Arabian sun for weeks at a time on pallets.

The service men and women drank them all day long. All of their symptoms are identical to aspartame poisoning. Dr. Roberts says "consuming aspartame at the time of conception can cause birth defects."

The phenylalanine concentrates in the placenta, causing mental retardation, according to Dr. Louis Elsas, Pediatrician Professor - Genetics, at Emory University in his testimony before Congress.

In the original lab tests, animals developed brain tumors (phenylalanine breaks down into DXP, a brain tumor agent). When Dr. Espisto was lecturing on aspartame, me, a physician in the audience and a neurosurgeon, said, "when they remove brain tumors, they have found high levels of aspartame in them."

Stevia, a sweet food, NOT AN ADDITIVE, which helps in the metabolism of sugar, which would be ideal for diabetics, has now been approved as a dietary supplement by the FDA. For years, the FDA has outlawed this sweet food because of their loyalty to MONSANTO.

If it says "SUGAR FREE" on the label - DO NOT EVEN THINK ABOUT IT!!!!! Senator Howard Hetzenbaum wrote a bill that would have warned all infants, pregnant mothers and children of the dangers of aspartame. The bill would have also instilled independent studies on the problems existing in the population (seizures, changes in brain chemistry, changes in neurological and behavioral symptoms).

It was killed by the powerful drug and chemical lobbies, letting loose the hounds of disease and death on an unsuspecting public. Since the Conference of the American College of Physicians, we hope to have the help of some world leaders. Again, please help us too. There are a lot of people out there who must be warned, "Please" let them know this information.

CHAPTER 8

ELECTRICAL BODY BOMBS

It could be argued that the most important system in the body is the immune system. The immune system is electrically indexed to the endocrine system. The endocrine system is a series of manufacturing plants that produce the chemicals and hormones and thus set up the electrical interface for many of the body's primary functions.

The immune system is the defense mechanism whose job it is to keep everything within the desired operating parameters. The immune and endocrine systems control our health more than any other systems in the body. Every part of our digestion has a downstream effect on our endocrine and immune ability. Every free radical (electrically disharmonious spent food particles and oxidized waste products of cell function), every piece of incorrectly digested food, every bit of toxic chemical we ingest puts stress on the endocrine/immune system function.

As the endocrine system starts to overload, it produces the wrong chemical, the wrong hormone, at the wrong time, in the wrong dose rate and for the wrong reason. The resulting imbalance then affects the electrical firing of the brain cell synopsis often inducing mood swings, anxiety, panic attacks, depression, chronic fatigue, PMS, etc. People then normally rush to their medical doctor who would, almost as a reflex action, reach for the prescription pad and scribble on it Prosac, or some other equally insidious drug.

One of the things that makes me really angry in my clinical work is when a parent brings me a young child that has been prescribed one of these designer drugs. Hyperactivity is usually the "disease" that the drug treatment is being used for. The child, by this stage, often seems like a zombie with no light in their eyes, no vigor, appearing lifeless. But as one mother said, "She is now very stable." I reminded the mother that dead is also VERY stable!

When you look at a young lamb running around the field full of life and vigor, it rarely does the same thing for more than two seconds at any time. One minute it will be lying peacefully resting. The next second it will be up bounding around the field, jumping joyously in the air. The next second it will be racing at full speed towards its mother, nearly knocking her off her feet, for a two-second suckle at the nipple, then off again at full speed in a totally different direction. This is natural young life.

Our grandmothers would have reacted to this similar normal childhood behavior with a... "Out of the house, you kids! Get out from under my feet and go and play somewhere else." The kids would have left the confines of the homestead and disappeared in all directions on the farm, playing in the water puddles, building huts, playing hide and seek and generally just burning up their natural, youthful vitality.

Today, the child is more likely locked in a one or two bedroom apartment, with limited outside playing areas and if there is one it is probably not safe without continual parental supervision. With this extremely limited opportunity to burn up their exuberant energy, amplified and distorted by the high levels of sugar and pop (aspartame) in their diets, and in a desperate attempt to be the natural young beings that they are, their behavior gets labelled as dysfunctional or hyper. Peace and quiet is not a natural behavioral pattern for the young lamb or the young child.

To force the child to fit the adult parameters of what is normal, the child is all too often given life-suppressing drugs. It is incredible that our society has lost so much knowledge of what it is to be a healthy, energy-filled child and to fit our twisted reality we too often attempt to drug the life force from our children.

However, there are times when a child's body gets slightly out of harmony, causing an environment that induces a population explosion of some micro organisms. For example: the child has a restless night's sleep and tosses and turns. She loses her blanket covering and her chest gets cold. Getting cold at night is one of the biggest triggers for "catching cold" or flu.

Colds and flu are not actually "caught;" they are a natural correcting function resulting from an improperly balanced biological terrain within the body, sometimes caused by the body's drop in temperature and the resulting pH change, but more often caused by the body's need to lower its general toxicity, to get the poisons out. The subsequent increase in temperature and mucus production is the body's natural way of dealing with the toxic loading.

Our modern reaction is to rush to the doctor for an antibiotic prescription or flu shot. We thank the doctor profusely while we give the child this life-killing substance which stops the body from doing naturally what it is meant to do.

Maintaining the body's biological terrain and a low toxic level is possible if the Ph is kept within its correct parameters. This can be assisted by drinking daily doses of apple cider vinegar, Grandma's hot tart lemon drinks, or taking adequate supplementation of electrically available formulations of Vitamin C, minerals, herbs and enzymes (refer to Appendix).

Oxygen therapy is also very beneficial (refer to Appendix). Many products and brands assist the cell oxygen uptake and scavenge the free radicals from the body, but look for the ones that are formulated from an electrical understanding, such as the products that are formulated with the new microcluster technology (refer to Appendix).

Keeping the bowels cleared with electrically available and electrically formulated natural herbal products (refer to

Appendix), can help correct the biological terrain of the bowel, maintain the body's Ph and lower any toxic build up. If the body and, in particular, the bowels are clean, the body does not need to "catch" a cold/flu to rid itself of the toxic overloads.

By suppressing the body's natural cleaning and detoxing process with the use of drugs we actually damage the immune system. The only way the immune system builds up strength and resilience is to naturally experience the factors that will trigger its response. This is well understood by the medical profession and is the basis for immunization.

However, immunization is an exceedingly different animal compared to the natural fortification process that occurs in the body. From an electrical perspective, what we call the disease is not the electrical imbalance the body originally experienced. The "chill" put the immune system under stress, allowing the subsequent microflora population increase. The body uses this increase to trigger a "spring clean." This "spring clean" we experience as the cold/flu. The "cold/flu" is the down stream physical display that an imbalance or toxic loading has already occurred. The "cold/flu" is not the "disease." It is the body cleaning and correcting itself.

Immunization ignores this train of events and in fact says the micro organism that the body is using to trigger its clean up "is the disease," and attempts to trigger the body to attack and kill that particular micro organism. The micro organism is not the problem, it was always meant to be there.

From an electrical point of view, immunization is based on an erroneous premise. Immunization is an electrical bombardment that has the effect of devastating the ability of the body to control its micro organism population naturally.

To inject, as in many immunization shots, any micro organism into the muscle tissue is a totally unnatural way for it to get into the body. It is impossible to produce in a laboratory that which millions of electrical interactions produce in our incredibly complex bodies. Not one of the micro organisms in an immunization shot contains the same frequency or the same electrical matrix of any micro organisms already existing in the body. So how can they accurately trigger the body's defenses?

The reality of immunization is that we willingly allow our children to be injected with disease-causing, toxic substances that produce dramatic and long-term electrical damage, that can manifest as many "diseases," including fibromyalgia, MS, malaise, hives, angiodema, allergic asthma, systemic anaphylaxis, Guillain-Barre Syndrome, encephalopathy, optic neuritis, brachial plexus neuropathy, many different types of paralysis, myletitis, polyneuritis (including cases of polyradiculitis, polyradiculomyelitis and polyganglioradiculitis), ataxia, respiratory infections, gastro-intestinal problems, eye problems, allergic thrombocytopenia, disturbed blood pressure, collapse etc. and other nerve and auto-immune system malfunctions.

As immunization is injecting or ingesting a totally foreign substance into us, this foreign substance, by being electrically incompatible, can only be perceived by the body as a poison. This is the cause of the toxic shock syndrome that sometimes accompanies immunizations. The micro organisms contained within the immunization shot may appear as the same species under a microscope, but once again this is not taking into consideration the specific electrical matrix (microscopic viewing does not show electrical function) of each organism and the interface it has with our electrical body.

The germ theory of disease stems from the research of a Frenchman called Louis Pasteur, but the true researcher in Pasteur's institute was the eminent scientist called Antoine Bechamp. Bechamp, the man without the public savvy, argued all his life that disease was caused by disharmony and imbalance of the body's natural microflora, but his boss Pasteur, being funded by his friends in the rapidly growing pharmaceutical industry, promoted the reality that bacteria caused disease and that bacteria could be killed by drugs.

Our entire germ-based micro-organism-killing pharmaceutical industry grew from this erroneous scientific premise.

It was Pasteur himself, on his deathbed, who apologized for deliberately taking Bechamp's research out of context, so that his institute could benefit from the funding that was coming from the newly emerging drug companies. In fact, he honored Bechamp with the correct scenario.

By then however, the drug companies and their "kill the germs at all cost" system had become entrenched and today, our health care system is a direct legacy of this lie (see the original research writings of Pasteur and Bechamp or the books, "Pasteur Exposed" by E. Hume and "The Dream Lie of Louis Pasteur" by R.B. Pearson).

Historically, there is evidence that suggests immunization is ineffective. Smallpox, Polio and all other diseases whose demise has been credited to immunization, were in fact on their natural downward trend prior to the start of immunization. As Smallpox and Polio immunization was started, the downward trend of these two diseases levelled off and actually started to go up again. In the case of Polio, immunization gave many people the disease. If left to run its own natural course, the disease would have been at an all-time low years earlier.

According to the British Association for the Advancement of Science, childhood diseases decreased 90% between 1850 and 1940, paralleling improved sanitation and hygienic practices, well before mandatory vaccination programs. Infectious disease deaths in the U.S.A. and England declined steadily by an average of about 80% during this century (measles mortality declined over 97%) prior to vaccinations.

If we look at the incidence of Rubella (German Measles), the greatest number of teenage girls who suffer from this so-called disease are those who have been immunized against it. To be immunized against Rubella increases the risk of having a physical outbreak because the immunization is introducing an electrically disharmonic, different and crude Rubella micro organism into the body.

There is no way that this Rubella organism is electrically anything like the one that could manifest in the body. To be artificially grown outside the body would cause its electrical frequency to be of a different electrical construct. This distorted and mutated "Rubella" then becomes the "disease," because the body has never seen or experienced it and has no defenses against it. Often the subsequent "catching" of the disease is the body's way of ridding itself of this toxin.

However, this still leaves the body open to any naturally occurring Rubella. Immunization introduces into the body something totally foreign, causing an electrical fry-up resulting in immune system damage. This leaves the body open to future attack from Rubella and other problems, particularly joint diseases.

The sad thing about childhood immunization, particularly Rubella, is that it often moves the "disease" from a relatively harmless childhood one to many more severe and devastating problems later in life including birth defects and miscarriage.

The HEW reported in 1970 that as much as 26% of children receiving rubella vaccination, in national testing programs, developed arthalgia or arthritis. Many had to seek medical attention and some were hospitalized for rheumatic fever and rheumatoid arthritis. (Science, US, March 26, 1977)

As with mumps, the incidence of rubella has shifted to older age groups since the widespread vaccinations for rubella. During the period between 1966 and 1968, 23% of rubella cases occurred among persons 15 years or over. In 1987 this same age group accounted for 48% of cases. (MMWR, Rubella and congenital rubella syndrome - United States, 1985-1988. 1989, #38, pp. 173-178)

A vast number of children who were injected with measles vaccine between 1963 and 1968 in the United States are now subject, as young adults to what is called "atypical measles." This is a very severe form of the disease in which it now appears that, because of the vaccination, there is an increased susceptibility to measles viruses, resulting from a damaged immune response. (JAMA, 1980, Vol. 1244, No 8, pp. 804-806)

A review of 1600 cases of measles in Quebec, Canada, between January and May 1989, revealed that 58% of school-age cases had been previously vaccinated. (MMWR, Measles - Quebec. 1989, #38, PP 329-330)

The same thing happens with the flu vaccines. Each year we are told to get the "shot" for the newest strain. The problem is that the "newest strain" was the one that was injected into us last year and caused a toxic loading. In its mutated and electrically distorted form it was able to survive in our body and mutate again.

In our bodies attempt to rid itself of this toxin we "caught" a cold or mild flu and then we spread it around with our breath until it took hold in someone with a low immune system, mutated slightly again, multiplied and came back to us as the "new strain." This process takes six to twelve months. Hence the six or twelve month recommended shots.

The only way to guarantee ever more flu strains is to keep on vaccinating. What a wonderful money making idea, never mind the continual hammering of our immune system in the process.

A well known flu epidemic - the "Spanish Flu" of 1918-22 - killed a large percentage of the healthy young male population in western Europe. This was the result of the American soldiers being vaccinated with flu shots prior to leaving for Europe and the first world war. The vaccinated soldiers mutated the flu in their bodies and with every breath and sneeze spread it throughout Europe. More young males died of the Spanish Flu than were actually killed in the theater of war. Vaccinations proved to be a far bigger and more deadlier weapon than anything the Germans threw at the allies.

A similar scenario has developed since the Gulf war with the American soldiers suffering "Gulf War Syndrome." This, in my view, is the electrical damage their bodies are suffering as a result of the extremely toxic vaccination shots they received prior to leaving for the Gulf coupled with excessive amounts of pop (Diet Coke, Pepsi, etc.). The pop contained Aspartame that when stored in the hot desert sun converted into wood alcohol which then devastated the electrical circuitry of the soldiers.

There are many reported cases of deaths soon after flu shots, from flu. Our immune system can only take so many hits. Also toxic shock resulting in death from "shots," is far more wide-spread than most people realize. The medical establishment works hard to keep the truth from being public knowledge.

The U.S. Federal Government's National Vaccine Injury Compensation Program (NVICP) has paid out over $650.6 million to parents of vaccine-injured and killed children, a rate of close to $90 million per year in taxpayer dollars. It is interesting to note that insurance companies (who do the best liability studies) refuse to cover adverse vaccine reactions.

In 1998 there was an article in the Vancouver Sun about the death of a teenage girl in Ontario, Canada. The article mentioned that she died of meningitis a week after she had been vaccinated against it. The article had not related the injection of the deadly poison as the cause of her death (or was it deliberately not being talked about by the medical "profession?") This could be considered a classic case of immunization-induced or toxic shock death.

To inject into the tissue any potentially life-threatening and toxic substance has to run the risk of causing a toxic shock effect. This is statistically known to kill three percent of its recipients. However, in truth the figure is very much higher. Recently, in a medical clinic where I work, a lady suffered a serious life-threatening emergency that lasted in excess of eight hours as a result of toxic shock induced by a flu vaccination given at another clinic less than an hour earlier.

It is also very difficult for a mother to come to terms with the death of a previously perfectly healthy baby within days, and sometimes within hours, of childhood immunization shots. Medically, the three percent death rate resulting from immunization shots, falls within the "acceptable risk" category. Ask the parent who has just lost their child as a result of childhood immunizations whether this is an "acceptable risk?"

Quote from the testimony of Michael Belkin, before the Advisory Committee on Immunization Practices, February 17, 1999, Atlanta Georgia:

"My 5-week old daughter, Lyla Rose died within 16 hours of her hepatitis B vaccination, which she received because of the universal vaccination policy this committee instituted in 1991. At her death Lyla had four of the eight highest-reported symptoms in the vaccine adverse reactions data. The NY Medical Examiner observed brain swelling at the autopsy, but refused to record that or mention the vaccination Lyla received in the autopsy report...

I hold each one of you who participated in the promulgation or perpetuation of that mandated newborn vaccination policy personally responsible for my daughter's death and the deaths and injuries of all the other beautiful, healthy infants who are victims of vaccinations . . .

For this government to continue to insist that vaccination adverse reactions reports do not exist is negligent, unethical - and is a crime against the children of America . . .

It is a sad day for the US when the nation's children need protection from the official medical authorities who are charged with protecting them from disease."

One of the most laughable scenarios is that some schools refuse entry to those children who have not been immunized. The reasoning behind this ruling is that the un-immunized children's disease-carrying potential is a threat to the remainder of the children. Surely, they are using twisted logic here. The very reason that most of the children were immunized was because of the belief that those children who had been immunized would not now be susceptible to the disease.

According to the above scenario, if there was an outbreak then surely it would only be the un-immunized children that would be at risk. The immunized ones would be safe, would they not???

If any school or kindergarten gives immunization as a condition of entry, just ask the school district or governing body to supply you with a written statement that if you vaccinated your child to fulfill their entry requirements, they will take full and unequivocal responsibly for any and all "adverse vaccine reactions." No insurance company in the world will cover "adverse vaccine reactions" - the risk is to high - so your school district will run for cover and the entire "entry problem" will cease to exist.

Some years back, in my search for answers to this whole immunization question, I had the opportunity to visit a play group that was attended by one to four year olds. I positioned myself where I was able to have an overview of the outside playground and there I observed and noted each child's behavioral patterns. I ranked each child's physical vitality, speed of movement, and observed their mental dexterity.

After an hour's observation and subsequent note taking, twenty one of the group had a relatively similar score but the remaining three scored very much higher than the main group.

At the parents' coffee break at the end of the play group, I approached the mothers of the three exceptional scoring children and asked them if they had immunized their children. Each of the three mothers answered that they had not. Upon further investigation of the group, I found they were the only three children attending that had *not* been immunized.

My belief, based on years of clinical experience and observation, is that the electrical bombardment due to immunization can have a profound adverse effect on our health and vitality that we can sometimes carry into adulthood. If the body is able to function in perfect electrical harmony without its immune system being destroyed by incorrect nutrition, doctor- or food-induced chemical poisoning and toxic bombardment, the strength of its own immunity is the best defense against disease states developing.

To ensure the body's perfect harmony from the beginning, breast feeding of infants for as long as physically possible is of extreme importance. It is also highly recommended to keep children free of chemically altered food and allow them to fully interface with soil and natural environments, i.e. allow the child to crawl around in the dirt and ingest a bit of soil, so that their body hopefully gets some natural bacteria to fortify their system.

To inject deadly poisonous and toxic substances into our infants is diabolically stupid at best, and at worst, an act of absolute barbarism.

It is not without reason that in some Asian countries, who have a greater understanding of the electrical componentry of the body, infant immunization is largely outlawed prior to two years of age. They perceive the infant's immune system is not strong enough to handle the possible toxic effects of immunization. In most western countries it is almost law that immunization has to be carried out *prior* to two years of age. When we look at the disease structure of the two different societies, disease in the western world far exceeds that of these Asian countries.

In 1975, Japan raised the minimum vaccination age to 2 years. This was followed by the virtual disappearance of cot death (crib-death) and infant convulsions. Then in the 1980's Japan (under pressure from the pharmaceutical companies) *allowed 3 month and older babies to be vaccinated; the incidence of cot death has increased again. (Vaccination, Viera Scheibner, PhD.)*

A study by the Center for Disease Control and Prevention in Atlanta, revealed a 2.7 times increase in seizure rates within four to seven days of the MMR shot and an increase of 3.3 times within 14 days. (What Doctors Won't Tell You, December 1995)

A comprehensive study of an immunization program of Kindergarten to 12th grade students revealed a 90% occurrence of the disease in those who received the vaccine. (New England Journal of Medicine, Vol. 320, 1989)

A large epidemic of diabetes (80% increase) occurred in New Zealand following a recent Hepatitis B immunization program and research scientists believe the most likely explanation is that the immunization program caused the diabetes epidemic. (New Zealand Medical Journal, May 1996, p 195)

Two-thirds of 103 children studied who died of SIDS (sudden infant death syndrome - cot/crib death) had been vaccinated within the last three weeks, many dying within a day of vaccination. (Dr. William Torch, Nevada School of Medicine)

When childhood vaccination rates dropped in Australia by 50%, SIDS also dropped by 50%. (Pediatric Supplement, Doctor's Forum, 1988)

Following the introduction of compulsory immunization, the incidence of diphtheria <u>increased</u> by 39% in France, 55% in Hungary, it trebled in Switzerland and increased from 40,000 to 250,000 in Germany, mostly affecting immunized patients. On the other hand, in Sweden, diphtheria virtually disappeared without any recourse to immunization. (Trevor Gunn, Mass Immunization)

The greatest threat of childhood diseases lies in the dangerous and ineffectual effects made to prevent them through mass immunization. (Dr. Robert Mendelsohn)

Immunization shots contain viruses and bacteria that are grown in pig or horse blood, rabbit brain tissue, dog and monkey tissue, chicken and duck eggs and calf serum.

This production system produces foreign (non-human) protein antigens that cause the electrical chaos in the human body. It is generally acknowledged that any foreign substances, such as in immunization shots, that have not been filtered through the body's normal digestive processes, can be highly toxic when injected into the muscles, lymphatic and blood systems.

Some foreign additives also normally found in various vaccines include:

* formaldehyde - a known carcinogen
* thimerosal - an organomercurial antiseptic, which is 49% mercury
* aluminum potassium sulfate
* aluminum phosphate - also used in deodorants
* lactalbumin hydrolysate
* phenol (carbolic acid) - extremely toxic
* acetone - volatile and can easily cross the placental barrier
* glycerin - tri-atomic alcohol derived from decomposed fats which can damage the kidneys, liver, lungs, local tissue (that's the cell damage at the injection site) and can cause diuresis and possible death.

And we willingly allow these toxic and dangerous substances to be injected into the flesh and blood of our babies and ourselves.

Immunization in all its forms, for whatever reason, is bombing the body's immune system. It has not gone unnoticed that the destruction of the immune system of the people of Northern and Central Africa has taken place since the World Health Organization went in and started mass immunization in the seventies. In fact, the advent of AIDS (which is an immune system failure with resulting viral attack) that some commentators claim originated in Africa, only became evident after this wide-spread and repeated immunization program.

In fact, AIDS is very different electrically from anything "nature" has produced. When I look at the energy that is AIDS, it is plain that natural evolution could not have developed a virus with such a remarkable selectablity that makes people with black skin pigment extremely vulnerable.

No other virus debilitates or kills with such precise selectivity. Also, the mathematical epidemiology of the AIDS virus suggests that a large number of people had to be simultaneously exposed. Mathematically this could only be possible with mass and repeated implanted exposure as in a immunization program.

There is overwhelming and substantial credible evidence, based upon government documents obtained under the Freedom of Information Act, that shows conclusively that the US government or its agencies, bioengineered the AIDS virus by recombining a cow virus (bovine spongiform encephalomyelitis) and a sheep virus (virsna virus - which has no known cure after forty years of searching). The evidence shows this recombined agent was proliferated in the smallpox and hepatitis B vaccines, the very vaccines that were used in the African immunization programs.

These two vaccines were also used in government-sponsored vaccination programs carried out in the male gay communities in San Francisco and New York, the two cities where AIDS "broke out" in North America.

Was AIDS bioengineered by the U.S. to "solve" the African overpopulation and continuous, expensive famine bailout problem and to also "rid" American cities of the "big bad scourge," the homosexuals? The evidence would suggest it was and to that end a class action suit was filed on September 28, 1998 before a U.S. Federal Judge. The Plaintiffs allege that the U.S. Department of Defense was involved in the "creation, production and proliferation of the AIDS virus."

The critical document in this suit is one that contains a record of Hearings held on June 9, 1969 and July 1, 1969 before a U.S. House of Representatives Subcommittee that contains direct evidence of bioengineering, including the Congressional Testimony of the Pentagon.

Another of the "Body Bombs" that our society uses to destroy the immune system function is what would generally be termed as recreational drugs. LSD, Ecstasy, Hashish, Heroin, etc., have the effect of causing chronic circuitry damage to our electrical body. There are exceptions of course, due to various resilient parameters in different people, but normally drug users' bodies very seldom recover their pre-drug use vitality.

Often the electromagnetic energy fields around the body are so damaged that the physical body shows symptoms such as inability to concentrate, indecisiveness, lack of direction, mood swings and a greater requirement for sleep, as well as the skin losing its luster, slow healing to normal cuts and abrasions, loss of hair tone and sometimes the development of intense, bulging eyes.

This last symptom is a classic case of the crown chakra, or the part of the energy system that is at the top of the body, being damaged. This is more predominant when the harder, narcotic and psychedelic type drugs have been used repeatedly.

Energetically, a hard drug user is very easy to distinguish and even ex-users hold within their energy fields the damage for many, many years. In some ways, the body never fully recovers from hard drug use.

The devastation caused to the body's energy system by recreational drug use is sadly often duplicated with prescription drugs.

However, the rebuilding of the body is possible if the former user is prepared to invest in their own recovery by taking high levels of electrically available minerals, vitamins and some very specific electrically formulated herbal combinations. For every year that one has taken drugs the recovery to full vigor and electrical function within the body, if at all possible, would take in the vicinity of three months.

However, non-drug user recovery from the degeneration associated with our modern life style would be one month for every year, which is the normal accepted standard within the natural health industry. This shows that to rebuild the body physically and electrically from drug use is three times more difficult than rebuilding the body from the normal traumas and stress loading of daily life.

One of the biggest bombs by far that we could ever expose the body to is chemotherapy. Chemotherapy has the effect on our electrical system that could be compared to a string of Napalm bombs on a forest. There is very little alive or functioning in any way afterwards.

The statistical recovery of cancer sufferers who elect surgery and chemotherapy is frighteningly low. Cancer in the last forty years has had more money thrown at it, more so-called research hours allotted to it, with the least amount of success than any other single ailment. Cancer is still one of the biggest killers and one would think that after more than forty years of research and treatment that has gotten us nowhere, our medical system would accept the fact that it has to look in other directions.

Sadly, the opposite has been the case. Every time anybody in the world has come up with a new approach in an attempt to alleviate the horror of cancer, they have either been legislated out of existence or been belittled beyond belief.

The "War on Cancer," like the "War on Crime," and the "War on Drugs" should be seen as self-perpetrating industries and NOT as attempts to find solutions that would put them out of business.

One example is the Essiac fiasco that has been ongoing in Canada since the 1930's. Essiac is a combination of natural herbs, given to humanity by the Northern Canadian Indians. It has the most proven track record of alleviating cancer and dramatically lowering pain associated with advanced cancer that I know of. It has no known side effects and has been used successfully by thousands of people.

However, the selling and administering of this formulation, as a cure for cancer, is illegal. In fact, the thorough documentation of Essiac and its cancer reduction properties, in the book *Calling of an Angel* by Dr. Gary Glum, has been banned in the United States and Canada.

How any politician, medical industry personnel, or pharmaceutical company shareholder can have a clear conscience over this, and the many other deliberately suppressed natural treatments, is almost beyond belief.

The medical profession's line of attack for cancer is to load the body up with life-destroying toxic substances (chemotherapy and radiation), whereas the natural health industry works to assist the body to come alive in all areas.

It is an extremely strange concept to any rational thought process, that one would use the strongest life destroying drugs in the belief that by doing so, life would be enhanced.

The cancer establishment is fixated on damage control - diagnosis, treatment and basic genetic research - and is indifferent, if not hostile, to cancer prevention - getting carcinogens out of the environment. Another factor is the conflicts of interests, which are significant when it comes to the National Cancer Institute, but profound and overwhelming when it comes to the American Cancer Society.

In his book, "The Politics of Cancer Revisited," Dr. Samual Epstein goes into great detail on the conflicts between the American Cancer Society and the cancer drug industry, the mammography industry, the pesticide industry and other such industries.

According to Epstein, the outgoing director of the National Cancer Institute left that organization to go to the cancer drug industry (nice little drug industry pay off). Another NCI director in the 1970s left NCI to go to the American Cancer Society and from there to head up the fiberglass industry (fiberglass is a recognized carcinogen).

Epstein charges that the cancer establishment is misleading people into believing that it is spending a good chunk of its stashed away billions on prevention - which is untrue. Looking for high crimes and misdemeanors? Read Dr. Epstein's book.

In my clinical experience as a Vibrational Medicine specialist, cancer is very preventable and recoverable, particularly in the early stages of diagnosis before surgery is required. Once surgery has been undertaken, electrical reconstruction using advanced Vibrational Medical knowledge is almost a requirement for the body to be able to complete the healing process.

If this electrical reconstruction is not carried out, the recurrence of cancer somewhere in the body within five years is almost guaranteed. With the correct electrical work and a perfectly healthy natural diet, in cooperation with the input of mega doses of electrically available herbs, vitamins and minerals, the recurrence of the cancer is largely nonexistent.

Am I suggesting that cancer can be cured? If that means returning the body to its pre-cancerous state or in other words electrical harmony, my answer would be an unequivocal "Yes," based on my clinical experience.

With what is known in the natural health field, particularly in Vibrational Medicine, and by using electrically available and formulated herbs, minerals and enzymes in the right dose rates at the initial diagnosis of cancer, there is the potential to bring cancer into the extremely "curable" arena.

However, if the client has elected chemotherapy bombardment, the recovery and non-recurrence is exponentially harder to achieve. A good read on this is in "Questioning Chemotherapy" by Ralph W. Moss, PhD.

Electing to go the chemotherapy route is often the same as signing your own death warrant. The electrical reconstruction of the body's energy system using all that the natural health industry has to offer is sometimes not enough after chemotherapy. However, in my experience, the success rates are still "hundreds of percents" better than only going the "medical" way.

If we look at the increase in cancers of all types over the last thirty years we see that its increase has parallels with the increase in preserved, chemically altered and laced manufactured food, immunizations and pharmaceutical drugs.

The death rate from cancer has never been lowered by medical intervention, pharmaceuticals or radiation. As Dr. James Compton Burnett in the UK said, "Cutting off the apples does not keep the apple-tree from growing apples." If the medical profession will not tell us the truth, then surely it is about time we used our own God-given brains and common sense.

"Everyone should know that the 'War on Cancer' is largely a fraud."
Linus Pauling, double Nobel Laureate.

Electrically, cancer is a massive electrical malfunction caused by a toxic and/or chemical overload and in the long term preventative scenario, the only possibility for alleviating the cause is for every mother never to feed a child anything that does not contain nature's electrical matrix.

That would mean no sugar, nothing with an artificial coloring, artificial sweetener, preservative, or anything that has in any way has been changed from the way nature intended. In other words, anything out of a packet, tin or that has been processed will contain within it an electrical matrix that has the potential to cause the electrical malfunction within the body that can manifest as the disease we call cancer.

Cancer is not something we "catch," cancer is one hundred percent self-induced.

The cause of cancer is simply the repeated electrical bombardment of the body from the toxins and chemicals we have injected or ingested. One of the most insidious electrical bombardments (toxins) we can give ourselves that adds to the risk of cancer is holding onto our emotional issues, allowing ourselves to be emotionally tight, holding on to a lot of judgments, blaming everything on everybody else and thinking the world has given us a bad turn. Cancer, is our own stupidity.

The medical profession as we know it today will never make inroads to alleviating cancer unless it is prepared to let go of its arrogance and the pandering to the multi-national drug corporations. They need to start looking at the electrical interface and the electrical damage that is the real cause.

Cancer is an electrical problem caused by toxins and poisons in our environment and can only be fixed, alleviated and "cured" from an electrical understanding. Perhaps the biggest single reason that this electrical understanding has not been taken on board by the medical profession is that nearly sixty cents in every medical dollar gets spent on our existing cancer scenario.

Therefore one could justifiably claim that cancer is too good of a "business" to be "cured."

Even though North America is ruthless in its suppression of anything that vaguely deviates from the gospel according to the "drug" industry, there are some countries that are starting to wise up to electrical truths pertaining to disease.

I copied the following from a display in the Schweiz National Science Museum, in Lucerne Switzerland. I quote!

"Electromagnetic Vibration.
How our cells communicate.
All healthy cells in the body can receive and communicate vast amounts of information in the form of ultra fine electromagnetic vibrations.
Along with vibrations in the natural environment (sunshine, for example) they shape all the body's biological processes. Techniques such as acupuncture and homeopathy have shown that a communication block between cells, rather than biochemical disorders, is often the cause of illness.
From this point of view, the increasing concentration of artificial waves in the environment is bound to cause problems. Radio, radar and microwaves effectively "jam" the exchange of information between cells, and so may provoke illness."

The above quote, approved by some of the world's foremost scientists for public display in a Science setting of this standing, had a profound affect on me. It validates everything I have been trying to educate people about. It validates fifteen years of my work and the reason for this book.

This scientific statement shakes the very foundation of our present medical belief structure. It is the first public scientific statement I have seen that rebuffs the decades of misinformation used by our drug-based medical system derived from the admittedly incorrect Pasteur theory. As the statement says, "vibrations shape **all** the body's biological processes."

Vibrations that the body cannot recognize as natural - those that did not evolve as part of nature - also shape the body's biological process. Toxic chemicals and pharmaceutical drugs, immunizations, manufactured food, chemical food coloring, artificial sweeteners, pesticides, herbicides etc., all contain unnatural vibrations. Likewise, artificial waves not only include radio, radar and microwaves, but also cell phones, X-rays, CT scans, ultrasound and all other frequencies (waves) that in its inherit wisdom, science and our modern civilization has bestowed upon us.

In the *European Court of Human Rights* on August 25, 1998, in the case of *Swiss Association of Electroapparatuses for Household and Industry* (FEA) versus *Hertel*, the Swiss Federal Court withdrew its verdict against Dr. Hans Ulrich Hertel. This case was reported in *The Journal of Natural Science*, Volume 2, No. 3, January - April 1999. Dr. Hertel was originally sued because he had stated that microwaves cause cancer. In an article published in the *Franz Weber Journal,* 1992, he wrote "that food prepared in microwave ovens damages health and leads to changes in the blood of consumers and said changes point to a morbid disturbance which could be the beginning of a cancerous process."

This European Court judgment spelled a severe reprimand of the Swiss Federal Court who had unanimously and without public trial issued judgment in favor of the *Swiss Association of Electroapparatuses for Household and Industry*

(FEA), against Dr. Hertel. The European Court after calling experts from throughout the scientific community passed judgment that the Swiss Court was wrong and after all the evidence presented to it, stated that Dr. Hertel was right and overturned the Swiss Federal Courts judgment against him. The Swiss Federal Court then issued a proclamation that all public restaurants who use microwaves must inform, by public signage, that microwaves may be in use in that public establishment. The Swiss Health Department also issued a general health warning against the use of microwaves.

It is generally public knowledge in many European countries that microwaved food is a health hazard, and in fact the production and sale of microwave ovens in Europe is grinding to a halt. It is incredible that in the United States of America very few people seem to be aware of the risk of microwaves.

Is it any wonder that we have effectively "jammed" the exchange of information between cells, and ***provoked*** illness. In Chapter Two I talked about the ten million two-way electrical transmissions that take place in the transformation of food to energy in our bodies, and how any disturbance to this transmission, this communication, is the start of disease.

As the body is an electrical reality, every aspect of every function is an electrical transmission, an electrical communication. To compromise (jam) any of these electrical communications is *"disease."*

The energy communication that takes place between every frequency of energy in this cosmos, and thus between human beings and each cell, is a scientific truth. "Traditional" medicine ignores this truth. But just as Gallileo was condemned to death for challenging the scientific truths of his day, it was nonetheless true that the Earth was round and circled the Sun.

Sadly, it was three hundred years after Gallileo died that the rest of the so-called scientific community took their heads out of the sand, threw away their blinkers, saw a different truth and discarded their own stupidity.

The electrical reality of the body and our ability to interface from a conscious level with the energy that we all are, may well be beyond the belief parameters of some. However, although Gallileo's peers had difficulties with their belief parameters, he was nevertheless correct. I hope those who cannot accept an electrical universe at this stage do not wait three hundred years to catch up to what is already known.

Help us get this information out

You can do this by recommending your friends and family to purchase this book, or even buy extra copies and give it to them as presents. We can only continue to do the work and research by having sales of this book. Thank you for supporting us in this manner.

CHAPTER 9

BIRTH'S ELECTRICAL TRAUMAS

During my years' of clinical experience, I have had countless hundreds of children brought to me with symptoms ranging from asthma to spina bifida. Specializing in Vibrational Medicine and being referred to as the "Body Electrician," the electrical cause of childhood disease states has always been of special interest to me.

With my experience of working with the body's electro-magnetic energy system I am able to follow the energy matrix of the disease backwards to the original trauma. In many cases, the electrical problem started years before. It took that long for enough cells to be electrically damaged and for enough circuits to "blow their fuses" before the problem manifested as the physical disease.

There is not a "disease" state that does not show up on the body's electro-magnetic energy fields prior to the physical manifestation of the disease. We are an electrical apparatus and the frequency that we vibrate at gives us the perception of our physicality.

Electro-magnetic frequencies of the body's system can be measured by using either extremely expensive scientific equipment, or, as we are also energy, we can teach ourselves, or be taught, how to be aware of vibrating frequencies of energy and bring that awareness to our consciousness - not unlike bringing some of the information contained on our computer hard drive onto the screen.

Therefore, to tune in, to become consciously aware of, communicate with and surf, as it were, the energy of another human being, is very much a learned art or diagnostic tool for those who are prepared to put in the time and effort. Once you have mastered this ability, the root cause of disease manifestations becomes very much easier to ascertain.

Our present medical model has absolutely no way of figuring out the train of events that lead to the physical manifestation of the problem. A trained Vibrational Medicine Practitioner is able to have an electrical communication with the energy fields of the body. Through this communication, it is possible to follow the frequencies back and be consciously aware of when and how the original trauma took place. This is how I am able to trace childhood disease symptoms back to the trauma that originally caused the electrical malfunction which years later manifested as a physical ailment.

Probably ninety percent of all childhood physical problems can be traced back to three major incidences in the life of the young child. The first factor, and possibly the most predominant one, was the way the infant was treated immediately upon its birth. The second factor is the severe electrical shock resulting from immunizations, and the third would be the effect of antibiotics.

I was fortunate that for the first forty years of my life I interfaced on a daily basis with animals. From my early twenties I was responsible for overseeing the births of up to five hundred cows annually. If you like, I am an extremely experienced midwife.

The reproductive system of that wonderful bovine, the domestic cow, is practically identical to the human reproductive system. In fact, all of the artificial insemination, in vitro fertilization, female egg extraction, fertilization and replanting techniques that are now used as relatively common practice in assisting women to become pregnant, resulted from knowledge gained in the dairy industry.

The New Zealand dairy industry leads the world with its fertility knowledge, which is the benchmark by which medical science sets its standards. As I lived and breathed this industry, I am very aware that to have a cow with calving difficulties usually meant that she was not able to come onto full lactation as quickly as one who did not, so it was extremely economically advantageous to have the cows calving naturally with the least amount of problems.

After twenty years or so of assisting in difficult births on the farm, I was able to see the difference in behavior of the mother and its young resulting from a difficult birth, as compared to those with natural, trouble-free births. There were many times when I have assisted with a difficult birth and the mother has subsequently totally rejected her young. Yet, in a natural, unassisted birth a rejection by the mother of its young is extraordinarily rare.

It was this observation with cows that led me to look at some of the problems that existed with mothers and children who ended up in my clinic. I initially started to question each mother who brought in an ill child about their birth experience and the subsequent immediate post-birth treatment of the child.

It soon became glaringly obvious that the greater the childhood disease state that had manifested, the greater the disharmony the child had suffered immediately post birth. Also, the mother's post birth depression could be traced to the disharmony experienced straight after birth.

Once I had established this physical correlation I then looked at the electrical matrix of the child's energy system to trace the physical symptom back to the electrical malfunction and then back to what caused the electrical malfunction. At this point a frightening discovery became abundantly clear.

In nearly every case of childhood asthma, allergies and many other health problems, the energy circuits that govern lung function were "blown out" as a result of doctor induced traumatic shock. This shock, in every case, was the result of a doctor's extreme physical abuse which was in the form of the proverbial "smack on the bottom" when the infant first came out of the womb.

This physical battering, done by any other person at any other time in one's life, would be classified as assault and would carry severe penalties, in some countries a jail sentence. Why is it that doctors can physically assault an extremely sensitive young being and not be aware of the absolute horror, shock and torment that young being must feel? Is it that our medical professionals are so diabolically naive to believe that a newborn child is incapable of feeling and reacting to any extreme stimuli?

This assault would have the same effect, when one looks at the electrical damage that occurs, as an adult whose car gets out of control and goes over a hundred foot bank and crashing down and hitting all sorts of rocks and trees on the way. The person survives the crash, but, as you can imagine, there would be serious psychological and emotional disturbances as a result of the trauma.

The electrical circuitry damage would also be great and would cause many downstream physical problems. Quite frankly, such persons would have been terrified out of their minds and their bodies would be in shock for days, if not weeks, after the accident.

To put a newborn infant deliberately through this degree of trauma is totally unacceptable and unnecessary in any situation.

To physically hit a newborn within moments of birth is assault and should be treated as such.

The reasoning given for this physical battering is that doctors believe it is required to start the breathing process. Well, excuse me Mr. Doctor, would you please tell me how every animal and every human being was able to survive and start breathing since time began prior to you getting your so-called education?

The entire modern birthing process that is carried out in most hospital situations is diabolically abusive to both mother and child. I have been called to assist many mothers in their birthing process and as a result have seen the amazing difference in the child's behavioral patterns and subsequent health, as well as the mother's emotional state, resulting from the immediate post-birth being traumatic or non-traumatic.

It is my experience that hospital births have a greater adverse affect on mother and child than midwife-assisted or home births. I am a passionate believer in the dehospitalisation of the birth process in all ways.

Giving birth is not a disease and in no way should be treated as such.

From an electrical understanding, I have never been able to find any residue trauma in the energy fields of the newborn as a result of the experience the fetus went through travelling the birth canal. However, during this part of the birth, the mother can sometimes experience extreme anxiety and discomfort. Any disharmony or trauma the fetus may or may not experience is obviously instantaneously transferred to the mother's energy body. The infant, in every case that I have observed, actually emerges from the birth canal electrically perfect, as long as no intervention such as forceps are used to assist delivery.

Any traumatic frequencies and subsequent physical malfunctions happen to the infant as a result of its experience in this world. (Please note we are not talking about the blood transfer problems or chemical toxicity that can occur as a result of the mother's state of health, we are focusing here on the electrical reality of the birthing process.)

The experience the child has at the time of its birth is totally controlled by the human beings that are assisting at the birth. Natural parameters such as hot, cold, in a house, in the back seat of a car or out in the bush or a field, appear to have absolutely no adverse impact on the traumatic loading of the infant's energy fields. The only traumatic loading that occurs is as a result of the human interface between the infant and those in attendance, including the mother.

In a perfectly harmonious birth, the mother would have had completely free movement, would have been able to make all the choices and have been in control of who and what assistance she desired. At the final stages of birth, she would have chosen to be either upright, in a squatting position, or semi-sitting with her bottom and back supported on a bean bag, so that gravity would have offered its maximum assistance.

To place the mother on her back during the birthing process is to go against every way the body and nature works. Gravity would be trying to pull the baby down through the mothers back, often resulting in lower back pain for years. To be on her back may be beneficial to an attending doctor, but one would have to question why the doctor was telling the mother what should be and what should not. Who was having the baby, the doctor or the mother?

The mother, if she was given the environment that allowed her to feel safe and secure, and one that she felt in control of, would possibly never elect to give birth flat on her back. In fact, she would probably have an overpowering urge to move around, to sway and generally allow her pelvic structure to loosen and open. She would naturally position herself so that gravity would assist the birthing process.

As the child emerges from the birth canal (in the perfect scenario), the mother would have taken its body with her hands cupped around each side of the infant's chest and assisted the infant's final passage from the birth canal.

Relaxing backwards, onto the support of the bean bag, for example, she would have drawn the infant up onto her hot, sweaty, very damp and bare breasts. There, for a moment, with skin to skin contact between the infant and the mother's breast, and skin to skin contact between the infant's back and the mother's hot hands, both mother and child would have rested.

The physical environment the child is now experiencing is as close as possible to the environment it has just left and knows so well. With its head buried into its mother's bosom it is aware of the mother's heartbeat which is so familiar. The wet and warm skin to skin contact is barely distinguishable from that of the embryonic fluids. The child feels safe and secure by the fact that it is cradled on one side by the mother's bosom and stomach, and on the other side by the mother's hands which are all but covering it.

If you can imagine for a moment that you spent nine months in a tank of warm water and the pressure of the water against your surface was the only sensation that your skin knew. Suddenly, without warning, you were extracted from that water, your life-giving umbilical cord was cut, you started to suffocate, you were held up, twisted around and then experienced a severe impact.

As you were lifted out of the water, the absence of any pressure against the skin would have made you feel as if you were expanding and about to explode. All of what you knew as your security - your life, does not now exist. You are instantly in a state of absolute terror and shock.

You would not dare move a muscle. You would be shocked into absolute rigidity. Unable to breathe and with no oxygen coming through the cut umbilical cord, you are rapidly turning blue and dying. The "doctor" swung you upside down (another traumatic experience, gravity pulling on your head outside the embryonic fluid), and fair whacked you on your behind! At that point you perceive your life as under total threat and you did the only thing possible, you screamed. The scream forced your lungs to prematurely start working, damaging the electrical circuitry (everybody smiles... except you!).

However, in the perfect scenario, nurtured on your mother's naked bosom, your body feeling the pressure of the skin contact, you felt safe and secure. You were not suffocating as you were getting all of the oxygen that you required, the same way as you had for the previous nine months, through your umbilical cord.

Slowly, you become aware of your different environment and as nature's impulses took over, you slowly moved your head. Your rested mother, responding to the same natural impulses, gently slid your warm moist body across so that your mouth came in contact with her nipple.

The electrical circuitry, or more correctly, the polarity between the top and bottom lip (the body's two most powerful circuits [meridians] - the governing and central, are connected to the top and bottom lips), connected with the electrical circuitry and polarity of your mother's nipple and the areola (the darker color skin around the nipple).

The resulting electrical connection caused an instant change in the mother's hormonal production. This allowed a physical stimulation in the cellular tissue of her mammary gland, and an electrical interface between the sphincter muscle in the nipple and the fluid contained within the mammary gland, resulting in the physical expression of the colostrum.

The infant, having an instantaneous reaction to stimuli from the warm colostrum, acted upon a natural instinct and searched for more (in fact, the natural instinct is once again a complex electrical process). As the infant's lips made repeated contact with the nipple and the areola, more colostrum flowed and the infant responded by suckling.

As the infant started to suckle and swallow, the electrical communication that was already taking place at the nipple allowed the lung meridian (circuit) to fire. This electrical connection caused the cells of the diaphragm, followed by the upper lobes, to start to expand and contract. Breathing started slowly and naturally as the electrical impulses to the lung circuit increased.

As the infant's body responded to the intake of oxygen through its own lungs, an electrical message was sent from the infant, back down its umbilical cord to the cells that connected the placenta to the inside of the mother's womb.

Contained within that electrical impulse was the message for the cells in the placenta to let go their attachments as oxygen was no longer required from this source. As the breathing increased, more electrical messages were sent to the placenta and greater numbers of cells unbuttoned until the placenta fully released itself from the inside of the mother's womb. The electrical instructions for the releasing of the placenta came from the now suckling and breathing infant, not from the mother's body.

To prematurely cut the umbilical cord, as is normal practice in most western hospital birthing situations, stops this entire electrical process from taking place. To cut the umbilical cord immediately after the infant emerges from the birth canal, is to cut its supply of oxygen instantaneously and stop any electrical messaging from taking place. The child becomes asphyxiated and subsequently immediately goes into traumatic shock (as you or I would if we were being suffocated).

The whack on the bottom, as you can imagine when you are hit suddenly and unexpectedly, causes a reflex action and the diaphragm spasms, which has the effect of taking in a quick sharp breath. This forced lung function prior to the natural circuitry connection, as mentioned above, causes severe damage to the lung circuitry. If this circuitry is not able to repair itself as the child grows, lung problems such as asthma are a guaranteed result. The predominance of lung cancer, even among non-smokers, could also be said to be directly related to this barbaric act.

Due to the umbilical cord being cut, the infant is unable to send the electrical messaging that is required for the releasing of the placenta. The placenta is a part of the baby and not a part of the mother's body. As the cutting and clamping of the umbilical cord stops the blood flow prematurely through the placenta, the placenta immediately starts to become toxic.

The mother's body recognizes this toxicity and goes into rejection mode which forces the unbuttoning of the placenta in an extremely electrically disharmonious fashion. She then expels the placenta from her body.

This sets up the scenario for the extremely widespread and insidious problem that mothers suffer called postnatal depression. This is a severe emotional imbalance and at times a life-threatening depressed state. It is very easy to understand, when we look at the birthing process electrically, that the cutting of the cord before the placenta was unbuttoned by the infant, forced the mother's body to go into rejection. This is a life-saving reaction on the part of the mother's body (if the placenta is not released quickly, severe toxemia may cause an extremely quick death for her).

The depression arises because the mother's body cannot distinguish between rejecting the placenta and rejecting the baby, due to the placenta and the baby being electrically indistinguishable. By rejecting the placenta, her body is telling her that the baby has been rejected also.

The resulting rejection mode that the mother's body goes into has a severe impact on her. On one hand, she is holding and looking at her newly born infant that she is meant to be madly and passionately in love with, and on the other hand, her body has gone into rejection. There is total electrical chaos. The mother's entire system can be blown out of harmony, leaving her in an emotionally devastated state. Nothing in her body will be functioning harmoniously and in fact the wonderful gift of breast feeding can become a nightmare. This is the reason for postnatal depression and the devastating trauma and guilt that many mothers experience after birth.

CHAPTER 10

ANTIBIOTICS and CANDIDA

With cesarean births, mothers often have rejection problems similar to those who have natural births, which can manifest as postnatal depression. However, there is the possibility of the child suffering even more so than the mother.

The devastating effects on the child's electro-magnetic system are amplified in C-section births due to the starvation effect that the child experiences as a result of the antibiotic bomb the mother was given prior to the cesarean. No hospital that I know of will operate without the cover of powerful and broad-spectrum antibiotics.

The mother's colostrum, sometimes referred to as the foremilk, contains live enzymes and bacteria that are essential to start the digestive process within the new-born baby's sterile stomach. Without this digestive process starting, the infant is totally unable to ferment any food, therefore causing the effects of starvation due to the child's inability to be nourished.

The antibiotic shot given to the mother will devastate the enzymes and micro-flora contained in her colostrum. When the baby suckles, it is getting a largely dead, unfermentable food. This will be experienced by the infant as extreme discomfort and stomach cramping similar to food poisoning.

This is why a large number of babies that are delivered by cesarean births lose weight dramatically post birth and do not appear to want, or to be nourished from, the breast. A high proportion of these babies end up being fed formulas. Their discomfort is recognized by extreme crying and as soon as the formula milk is introduced they settle and appear satisfied. This is because the formula milk contains some live enzymes and micro-flora which start the digestive process. However, formula milk is an extremely poor substitute for live colostrum and mother's milk.

One of the easiest ways mothers and midwives can overcome this problem is to use natural bacterias such as Latero Flora, Acidophilis Bifidis and other friendly floras mixed with natural yogurt and smear it around the nipple and inside the baby's mouth for all of its initial suckling attempts.

Also the mother can take up to three liters a day of this bacterial-laced natural yogurt for up to a week after her antibiotic shot. This will rebuild the micro-flora back into her system and with that the life giving aliveness of her breast milk.

The infant's stomach, by getting some of the correct gut bacterias from the "fortified" natural yogurt, will be able to start its digestive process immediately and thereby be nourished by the mother's milk without the need for artificial milk formulas.

I have personally, in a clinical situation, been able to see the dramatic positive results of this yogurt kick-start with cesarean birth babies. In these situations the baby's birth weight is surpassed within three days and the new-born loves the breast. Normally, the baby is totally content and never cries. This, for cesarean births, is relatively rare.

To deny a newborn infant nature's most potent food, by killing the colostrum's ability to be fermentable, and not rebuilding its aliveness and thereby its nourishment-giving qualities, is to my way of thinking, inexcusable.

I have had countless lambs and calves showing next to no signs of life, so near death the only physical movement they could manage was a slow blink over deeply sunken and dry eyes, yet when they were given a few ounces of warm colostrum, they have been able to hold their heads up within minutes and voice their demands for more. In fact, I have had lambs brought into the house so dead and cold that normally I would have elected not to feed them. But within minutes of syringing colostrum in to their stomach, they have been running around the farm kitchen. That is the power of live colostrum.

For many years now I have been advising a large number of my clients, in particular some cancer sufferers and others with severe digestive disorders and chronic degenerative diseases, to find a source of colostrum.

There is a source of Colostrum that we have now found and recommend. It is the only source of Colostrum available in North America that is from New Zealand pasture-fed outdoor living cows and it contains the most bioelectrical activity and it is dried from the liquid and powdered by the best technology in the world (refer Appendix under Colostrum). This Colostrum can be safely taken by newborn infants to the day you die. It contains nature's electrical matrix of pure food. It could be argued that this Colostrum may well be the best form of nourishment that we could possibly get other than our mother's milk. There are no over-dose limits and it can be taken by anyone at any time. **It is not milk.**

It was quite normal in the old days for the mother of a sick child to take that child to a neighboring farm and have the child suckle from the mother of a new-born. In those days there was always one mother in the community who had just given birth. It is quite normal for children into their early teens to be treated with colostrum in this way.

It has always amazed me that the medical profession has never embraced the use of bovine colostrum for the treatment of many of the common illnesses. Colostrum (bovine or human) is the most powerful life-giver or immune system rebuilder that is known to exist on earth. To treat cancer with extremely high levels of electrically available enzymes, electrically available friendly flora and herbs with the added input of high levels of Colostrum is nearly always successful. In fact to not treat cancer with the above is to have a death wish.

Colostrum can be mixed in with baby formula to supply the necessary colostrum components that are not contained in formula and that may also be missing from the mother's breast milk, due to antibiotic coverage during the birthing process.

Its good to see (and encouraging) that some sectors of the scientific community are catching up to what natural health practitioners have been saying for years.

Bacterial-enhanced natural yogurt is also very important in the rebuilding of the immune and digestive systems. There is a specialist natural yogurt manufacturer in New Zealand (refer to Appendix) who produces under license the world's first yogurt cultivated from the registered B.O.D. Strain of Bifidus bacteria (Supreme Flora/Flora Balance/Latero Flora) that many doctors are recommending for various childhood digestive problems.

This natural yogurt is without doubt one of the best natural health products for the rebuilding of the digestive system, particularly after antibiotic treatment or other digestive imbalance. Because it contains the B.O.D. Strain of Bifidus (a unique and very different natural bacteria) it is also one of only a few natural products that is truly effective in reducing the candida loading so prevalent in the world. Candida fungus causes insidious long-term health problems and is always the result of taking antibiotics.

Doctors not recommending rebuilding the intestinal flora with natural bacterial products containing the B.O.D. Strain of Bifidus (refer to Appendix) at the completion of an antibiotic treatment should face malpractice procedures.

The yogurt referred to above is made with exceptionally high standards of integrity and truly contains within it a frequency of energy and electrical compatibility with the human body that is extremely rare to find in any food. The energy contained in this yogurt is largely due to the fact that this plant is a specialist, family-owned and run operation and the frequency of love and honor is contained within the amazing foods they produce. Their products have been recognized within an extremely competitive industry with the awarding of many gold medals for their specialist cheeses and yogurts.

Antibiotics and their chronic overuse in our normal medical system is the second most devastating body bomb, after post-birth trauma, in its impact on the health of children. I have dealt with literally hundreds of children struggling with their health as a result of indiscriminate antibiotic use. It is my opinion that for a doctor to prescribe antibiotics, outside of a clearly life-threatening situation, should be cause for their dismissal as health care providers.

The use of even mild dosages of antibiotics by children totally devastates and kills a large percentage of the microflora contained in every part of their body. The resulting imbalance allows for a rapid unchecked population explosion of the naturally occurring candida fungus because antibiotics have no ability to kill candida. With a normal healthy bacterial population, candida is just one of hundreds of natural microflora and is therefore kept in its normal population context. The body bomb effect of antibiotics leaves this natural fungus with no checks and balances.

This candida problem can stay with the child into adulthood and is the underlying trigger for many, if not all, disharmonies and emotional problems developing in the body for years afterwards and possibly also later on in life.

As the candida population goes up, its need for food increases. The predominant food sources candida requires are sugar and gluten (a constituent of grain, particularly wheat). This is why many people with high candida loadings have cravings for sugar- and grain-based products. This then drives their subsequent weight gain. Sugar and bread/muffin/pasta cravings are very often an extremely definite sign that the microflora balance has become very distorted. To lower candida levels, **total** abstinence from sugar and grain intake is of paramount importance.

In order to rebalance the microflora in the system, it is necessary to reintroduce the natural bacterias. Many Natural Health Consultants have been recommending Acidophilis for this purpose. However, although this is beneficial, on its own it will not create the balance that is required. Acidophilis bacteria does not act as a strong enough pathogen fighter and thereby does not reduce the candida fungus count sufficiently. On its own it will simply not do the job.

With the latest scientific understanding and knowledge about stomach bacterias we can now use the newly found natural bacterias such as the B.O.D. strain of Bifidus (refer to Appendix) or other electrically available flora such as Friendly Flora (refer to Appendix), containing L. Salivatus and L. Plantarium.

When these bacteria are combined with Acidophilis, the required decrease in the candida loading is in most cases guaranteed. In fact, using the above bacteria, plus adhering to a strict eating regime that eliminates all sugar and all grain, is *the* most effective anti-candida program (It is suggested that you take the B.O.D. strain of Bifidus and the L. Salivarius / L. Plantarium combination at different times throughout the day to maximize their potential).

To use any candida control program that does not utilize the B.O.D. strain of Bifidus is, as far as I am concerned, to be naive to the findings of the latest scientific research. The B.O.D. strain is the most effective candida-killing natural bacteria to have been discovered. Its effectiveness is dramatically greater than Acidophilis, but the above combination appears to enhance the qualities of each and the combination is extremely powerful.

High candida loadings on our body's system could be seen as the single biggest trigger in the development of all childhood disease scenarios. In fact, taken outside the childhood parameter, candida is the biggest single infliction of non life-threatening health problems in the western world and is always the precursor for chronic fatigue. There are over two thousand physical symptoms attributed to candida imbalances and high candida levels are believed to be, by an increasingly large number of researchers, a major factor in the ever-increasing prevalence of cancer.

Candida growth explosion and subsequent massive symptomatic problems have been known to the top echelons of medical science since the mid 1950's. The medical profession has chosen to ignore the devastation to the human body as the result of this imbalance because antibiotics were believed to be the panacea for the human race's ills - no doubt helped by the fact that antibiotics were the leading profit makers for many years.

How then could the medical system own up to the fact that its most profitable product was the cause of nearly every disease that walked into their clinics?

Then again, it may have been that antibiotics were recognized as the king hit. Every time you prescribed them, you knew that the body's immune system would be further compromised, candida's population would explode, and even more disease would transpire. You had a winner, a never-ending stream of sick people, made sick by the perceived cure. The perfect and very profitable business.

Even though candida and its related symptoms are becoming glaringly obvious to the highest echelons of medical science, the mind set and the momentum that the antibiotic industry has generated for itself is an extremely difficult juggernaut to slow or have any hope of reversing.

Mothers often bring children to me suffering from multiple symptoms, such as chronic runny nose, repetitive earache, pastey-colored skin, chronic pimples, period problems, irritability, dysfunctional behavior, learning difficulties, antisocial behavior and just obviously looking as if they are struggling for survival. Upon questioning when the child had last been prescribed antibiotics, the mother, more times than not, with tears in her eyes, draws the latest antibiotic prescription from her purse. Knowing full well that antibiotics only added to the disharmony and misery in the child's body, the mother in desperation was seeking another answer.

Candida and its related symptoms are so easy to be seen by the trained eye. By looking at the energy field of the client, I can pick up and read the candida loading within minutes of the client being in my presence. One of the classical physical symptoms is redness around the upper and or lower eyelids.

Other symptoms are food allergies, reactivities, chemical intolerances and general inability to function in this modern world. These symptoms are always, always, associated with the antbiotic-candida-microflora imbalance.

Many people, especially females, relate candida to a narrow group of problems such as vaginal yeast infections but, in fact, yeast infections, athlete's foot, severe itchiness of the skin etc., are just a few of the many hundreds of candida symptoms.

It surprises me, the shocked questioning look I get from mothers and others when I categorically state there is no such disease as an allergy. Allergies are the physical symptom of the body's inability to correctly ferment and thus make electrically available the particular food that was ingested, or the body's inability to detox the environmental pollutants.

It is the body's reaction to the poisons or toxins produced or subjected to, that we call an allergy. Often it is possible to trace so-called allergic reactions, for example dairy intolerance, back to the destruction of the gut bacteria caused by antibiotics (in young children it can also be the result of the doctor-induced trauma mentioned earlier, blowing its system out). It is not the food product itself which is the cause of the allergy, but rather the fact that the child/adult does not have the correct biological terrain or electrical function necessary to break down or digest the food.

In my clinical experience, cesarean birth children have a higher incidence of allergies due to their stomach never receiving the full compliment of live colostrum. Add these antibiotic scenarios to the electrical bombing of immunization shots at six weeks of age and you could not create a better recipe for illness and disease if you tried.

These three body bombs - post birth trauma, antibiotics and immunizations - are the three things that I would suggest are creating a large portion of all illnesses we develop in our lives. The only way we will be able to increase our health and vitality is to remove the causes of our electrical malfunctions and stop treating the symptoms of these body bombs by stopping the bombing.

Due to the widespread damage to our electrical system, our immune system has been continually under stress since our childhood, and as we progress through our life our immune system is never able to obtain its full, correct function. The priority in rebuilding our health and vigor would be to rebuild immune function and microfloral balance. This rebuilding process can be done with correctly formulated and electrically available natural bacteria, enzymes, minerals and herbal supplementation.

Very often as we go about this rebuilding process, we will need specific electrical work done to our energy system by a particularly well-qualified and experienced Vibrational Medicine Practitioner.

One of the most profound self-help things any of us can do is to have adequate levels of available protein in our diet and to have more free movement, such as dance and childhood physical playing activities. Extremely physical and repetitive sports and gym workouts produce more toxins and stress in the body than are usually cleaned out.

Happy, joyous movement is by far the best "exercise." Free dance is definitely near the top of the list. Lymphacising (bouncing on an electrically tuned mini-trampoline, refer to Appendix) is the best detoxing lymphatic draining and immune system enhancing movement one can undertake. Good brisk walking is also extremely beneficial.

None of the above suggestions in isolation will do everything for you, but put together in balance they all add to the potential of each other, so the sum becomes very much greater than the individual components. This is the basis of Electrical Nutrition and Vibrational Medicine.

CHAPTER 11

ELECTRICAL CLEANSING

The first question most of us ask is why do we have to clean up our bodies? The easy answer is because we spend a lifetime gunking it up! Our modern food intake, particularly those foods that contain high levels of wheat and sugar, combined with our sedentary lifestyle, have the effect of slowing the body's natural cleaning systems.

Obviously the best way of cleaning the body is to start at the top. If we stopped pouring in the electrically distorted food, our systems might actually catch up in the cleaning departments. However, that would be an extremely slow process, and most of us would be dead as the result of the degeneration brought on by the level of toxic gunk within our system before that cleaning process was finished.

Many people are in such denial about the causes of their physical problems, they find it difficult to accept that a large percentage of everything that is going wrong in their body is the result of what passed between their two lips. It has been said many times that you are what you eat. There has probably never been a more truthful statement.

The biggest difficulty we all face is that, in most instances, we do not believe there could be any long term damage by eating the "average" diet. Hopefully you are now starting to realize that we may be prematurely killing ourselves. Our previously held beliefs, with regard to food, were based on completely erroneous premises and concepts.

By starting at the top, the obvious choice would be to have a large percentage of our food intake consisting of raw, fresh fruit and vegetables, accompanied by a far greater amount of crude protein to what we have been lead to believe is required, and a greatly reduced amount of grain and starches. The correct combinations, to assist the body in all its processes, would be to combine vegetables with crude protein or vegetables with carbohydrates, but never combine proteins with the carbohydrates in the same meal.

The benefits of good food combining are extremely noticeable, if you are prepared to be aware of how you feel and your subsequent energy levels when you change your diet. The heaviness and bloated feelings after a hearty meal do not exist with correct food combinations, which suggests the fermentation process is taking place within its correct parameters and thus you are not adding to the toxic loading of your system.

Now that we are not pouring the gunk in the top we had better break loose the toxic buildup that is in the lower digestive tract and bowel. There are many ways that we can approach this, the best being herbal formulations that have been electrically combined (refer to Appendix). However without adequate levels of hydration, the process will be slow.

Water that is able to electrically interface with our cells, or electrically alive water, is the biggest single requirement for this job. There is not one part of the body's system, physically or electrically, that can function in the absence of electrically alive water. The entire electrical function of every cellular process in the body depends on the electrical conductivity contained within every molecule. This conductivity increases and decreases depending on the hydration levels of the cellular structure.

We have been told that drinking water will increase the hydration of every cell within three minutes, but sadly this is not the case. The chemically-laced water we drink in today's cities and towns, even if we buy purified water or filter it ourselves (filtration takes out the dangerous toxic chemicals that the city council put in, but the water is still left electrically damaged or electrically dead), is unable to adequately hydrate our cells.

This lack of hydration happens because the surface tension of this water, due to the chemically-induced damage, is far greater than the surface tension of the body fluids that surround every cell. The electrical bonding of the molecules (surface tension) of our electrically damaged drinking water is such that the water is unable to electrically interface with our body fluids.

This is why when we drink a glass of water, we have to run to the bathroom within a very short space of time. Our body's elimination system was forced to dump the water immediately because it was unable to enter our body fluids. The water, in essence, was toxic to us because of its electrical incompatibility and therefore was not able to be used to clean and flush our body tissues. Hence the difficulty for many of us to detoxify our bodies effectively and control obesity, not to mention the extreme stress we have put our kidneys under.

This hydration issue was not a problem a hundred years ago when we drank the live water nature supplied us. However, since we have moved away from the streams, springs and wells out on the farm, we have been forced to utilize chemically-laced water that even with filtration, is so electrically damaged it is largely unavailable to us.

This water could be termed electrically "dead."

As a result of a life time of research, Drs. Patrick and the late Gael Flanagan, discovered a very simple and cost effective way of reducing the surface tension of water to make it electrically available, the way nature had originally supplied it to us, so it can actually be absorbed into our body fluids.

This new technology is termed "Microcluster technology" (refer to Appendix under Microhydrin) and is available in liquid or capsule form. By lowering the surface tension, it not only makes water more electrically available to our body fluids, but it also changes the electrical conductivity potential.

The scientific breakthrough by the Flanagan's is one of the greatest advancements in natural health in decades. We can now achieve the cleaning of the body and rehydration to levels previously unknown in our modern times.

No other products or processes are capable of achieving this because their electrical matrix will not allow that rapid interface with the cells. Firstly, the body has to separate the electrical matrix of the H_2O molecule from the different components in the drink before it is available for hydration. Your can of pop, your cup of coffee or even your glass of orange juice does not do the job. There are three rules to effective hydration. The first one is alive, electrically available water. The second one is alive, electrically available water. And the third one is, you got it, alive, electrically available water.

With a large part of our western society making their living by sitting in offices and using their brains, the requirement for hydration is exceedingly important because the brain contains a greater electrical complexity than any other group of cells in the body.

The only way the electrical body functions at a cellular level is through the conductivity of the fluids in and around the cells. Therefore, the hydration of the brain cells is the biggest single factor in attaining maximum brain function. Very often people that work with their heads could alleviate the tired and fatigued feelings just by increasing their intake of electrically alive water.

Working the body physically hard is usually accompanied by enhanced breathing. This increase in breathing will trigger the thirst alarm by drying the breath channels, including the mouth, and extremely quickly you will relate this to needing another drink. However, in mental work the trigger that we call thirst often does not fire because the increase in breathing, normally accompanying an increase in work, is not now happening.

Our change to a nonmoving lifestyle has been faster than the body's ability to adapt and provide us with another thirst signal. As hydration levels go down, so does our electrical function. Physically we are actually poisoning ourselves. We have to be consciously aware of this lack of physical stimulation for water and be disciplined to take regular drinks throughout the course of the day. To achieve adequate hydration for maximum brain function we would require a minimum of three liters of chemical-free, electrically-realivened water, taken over six to eight hours.

To recap... without adequate hydration levels in the cells there is not one electrical process that can be correctly undertaken in our body. Therefore the cleaning out of toxins, as well as having good brain function, regardless of how good our diet is, is an electrical impossibility if there is insufficient electrically alive water intake.

To those people who embark on a serious detoxing program, the water intake required over a twenty four hour period would be up to half a gallon of water the way nature made it, electrically alive.

Some of the symptoms of dehydration (poisoning) that we experience in our sedentary lifestyles are headaches, sleepiness, inability to concentrate, irritability, muscle tightness, constipation, acne, heavy watery eyes and general lethargy.

If you are sitting at your computer and become aware of any of these symptoms get up, have a two minute brisk walk around the office, drink two or three good glassfuls of electrically available water, and you will most likely feel alive again and your work output will jump.

The next stage in cleaning up the toxic loading is movement. Good cleaning detoxing movement is not going to the gym for a hard workout. Most gym-based physical workouts produce more toxins than the lymphatic system is capable of cleaning out. Gym-based workouts are predominantly designed to increase muscle strength and definition and that technically involves the stripping of muscle tissue which triggers a rapid cell reproduction. This is how muscle mass is increased.

The movement that is required for a detoxification process is the kind that drives the lymphatic pump without causing cell strip down. The lymphatic drainage system is a series of complex interrelated one way valves called lymph nodes. These valves govern the flow of lymphatic fluid. The flow of the lymphatic fluid is upwards from the feet towards the neck, then through the sub clavicle valve which returns the lymphatic fluid to the blood for cleaning and the elimination of toxins by the liver and kidneys.

From the cranial structure the lymphatic fluid drains down towards the neck. That is why the brain works best when we are upright, because gravity is taking care of the cell cleaning process, but the rest of our body needs to move downwards in order to drive the lymphatic fluid upwards against gravity.

This necessitates regular and repetitive, vigorous up and down movements of the body. The most efficient up and down movement, with the least cell strip down and carried out in an upright position to maximize lymphatic movement, is to bounce on a small (approximately thirty six inches in diameter) electrically tuned rebounder (mini-trampoline).

There are many mini-trampolines on the market, but I know of only one that has been electrically tuned to the electromagnetic frequency of the body's electrical system (refer to Appendix). This is so that the frequency it produces does not damage the body's energy system, as is the case in most commercially produced mini-trampolines.

An electrically tuned rebounder means the frequency that is generated, as a result of the bounce, produces a vortex of energy that is compatible with the body's electromagnetic energy field. The bounce generates a field of energy due to the fact that the nylon mat and the springs are being tensioned and then released. This "stress" of the mat and the springs changes the frequency within the molecules which relates to a force field of energy being generated. On a rebounder this energy field, or force field, is vortexed or spun by the outer metal band and its amperage can be up to a thousand times stronger than the human energy field. To have this generated field of energy (vortex) out-of-faze with the body's energy field creates a yucky feeling at best and an electrical distortion in the body's fields at worst. This is why many commercially available rebounders do not feel good, regardless of the salesman's blurb.

A group of lymphologists back in the eighties recognized this potential problem and many, many thousands of dollars was expended in the scientific research and recording of the frequencies of different springs, ratios and materials. As a result, over a five-year period, a very sophisticated electrically tuned rebounder was developed. The rebounder we refer to in the appendix is the only one in the world that we know of that has had this scientific research and tuning done to it. To the naked eye it may look the same or similar to every other one, but just as the model A Ford and the new Ferrari both have four wheels, an engine and breaks, one has had a lot more technology and tuning and they do the job very, very differently. The eye cannot see all things that are real. An electrically tuned rebounder is a very, very different machine to the commonly available rebounders and will not distort the body's energy fields in any way, in fact you will feel totally invigored and powered-up from even two or three minutes bouncing upon it. The technology actually does work.

This electrically tuned rebounder is probably the most important and profound health apparatus that any of us can use. Singularly, this machine will do more for our health than anything we could ever own.

The next most beneficial lymphatic drainage movement is that of brisk arm-swinging walking. Jogging actually produces about the same amount of toxins as the up and down movement is removing. It has been said, to take the shock out of jogging would be the best exercise on earth. Lymphacizing (using specific bouncing techniques on an electrically tuned rebounder) does just this.

Any other exercise over and above the jogging effort usually hinders rather than helps the spring cleaning efforts. Usually they produce more muscle mass and strength but do not necessarily enhance duration, and duration is the only indicator of fitness. Duration is also an indication of lymphatic system efficiency. Think about this next time you are about to rush off to the gym. However, going to the gym is certainly better than not doing anything.

If you do not have an electrically tuned rebounder or a gym membership and do not really want to go for a good brisk walk in minus fifteen degrees Celsius or plus ninety eight degrees Fahrenheit, then how about putting on your favorite music, some comfortable clothing and literally dancing your butt off.

If you spent the same amount of time per day vigorously dancing, as you would ideally spend in a gymnasium, I guarantee you will achieve a greater degree of lymphatic drainage and health improvement by doing so. In fact, to dance only requires your will to do it, no fancy leotards, no memberships, no cost structures or driving your polluting car to the gym. However, it is often easier to be disciplined to dance with some friends. So instead of the morning coffee meetings on your street or after-work drinks in the bar, how about a daily dance gathering? You will be a lot healthier and a whole lot happier.

Do not forget, ladies, your lymphatic drainage system has to move all the lymphatic fluid up through the lymph nodes that are contained in the outer connective tissue around your chest. To wear bras every waking moment goes against everything your body is trying to do to detox and reduce your cellulite. I am not suggesting that you burn your bras, but please, please do your exercises and spend some hours a day with minimal restriction around your chest. It has been suggested that the biggest cause of breast cancer is the restriction on the lymphatic drainage system due to long-term wearing of bras.

Most people do not realize that one of the only ways to reduce that unsightly cellulite on women and those extra inches of flab on the bellies of us men, is to move it out through the lymphatic drainage system. The other way to get it out is to self-induce a famine, or to it put plainly, starve yourself.

The only trouble with this latter approach, often referred to as fasting, is once food intake is recommenced, the body naturally responds by increasing its efficiency of food conversion, which is a natural biological response. As a result, lost cells are replaced incredibly quickly and this is why fasting achieves very little.

Fasting also produces extreme stress on various systems within the body, resulting in electrical system damage which can lead to disease. Looking at fasting from an electrical perspective, it becomes clear that there are far more effective ways of undertaking a detoxing process.

One of the more pleasurable lymphatic drainage processes we can avail ourselves of is massage. However, many massage therapists and teaching institutions have such a chronic lack of understanding of how the body is constructed that many of the massage strokes are carried out against the direction of the lymphatic flow.

The lymphatic system contains hundreds of extremely delicate non-return valves and to use a massage stroke that has the effect of forcing the lymphatic fluid against the natural opening of these valves has the potential to seriously damage their one-way function. For correct lymphatic drainage, all firm massage strokes, at all times, should go from the extremities towards the neck. This is undebatable and to be in denial of this knowledge or to choose not to use this knowledge, is to be dangerously ignorant.

As suggested earlier, the lower digestive tract and colon can become very toxic due to incorrectly fermented foods, and so cleaning the digestive tract is of paramount importance in any detox program. There is a tremendous amount of information regarding colon-cleansing techniques and processes, some of which necessitate the flushing of the colon by inserting tubes up through the anus (colonics).

When we look at how the body is physically constructed and in particular, the way the sphincter muscle controls the anal opening, it is very easy to see that the construction of this muscle is in the form of a one-way valve. The design is to allow movement from inside of the body to the outside. To feed any object from the outside in through the anal opening is to totally distort and electrically damage the cells of the sphincter muscle. Under no circumstances do I recommend colonic flushing because of this potential electrical damage.

Also, the inserting of the tube, in colonic flushing, has an extremely high chance of damaging another one-way valve system in the upper rectal cavity, the transverse rectal fold valve. These valve systems are electrically connected to the circuitry that governs the spasming of the levator anal muscle and other muscle groups within the rectum. Because they are also electrically connected to the upper colon cavities, the electrical damage to a large portion of the colon is a high possibility.

The follicles on the inside of the colon cavity send an electrical message down to the valves of the anus and control the opening and closing. Any damage to the electrical function of this complex circuitry has a possibility of promoting the onset of colon cancer. Remember cancer starts as an electrical malfunction.

Even though colonics are recommended as being one of the methods used to reduce the risk of colon cancer, the possible electrical damage may outweigh the benefits. The entire colon system is constructed for the one-way movement. Anything other than this one-way movement is an extreme violation of nature's complex plumbing system, as well as a total distortion of the electrical interface between millions of cells.

There are many other ways to ensure the buildup of semi-decayed matter is removed from our colon, but sadly many of them put the body under far too much physical stress, thereby causing electrical damage to massive amounts of cells within the colon. Any cleansing method that creates physical discomfort is electrical bombardment. Most drug-based diuretics fall into this category.

Many herbal concoctions can also have a powerful cleaning effect on the colon and, sadly, a large percentage of herbal-based colon cleanse formulations do not take into consideration the electrical chaos that results from their vicious action.

The object of the exercise is to move all of the digested food matter through the colon as well as slowly softening and removing any built-up residue on the walls of the colon. At the same time, it is necessary to supply to the cells the nutrition needed to help rebuild any damage.

A successful, trauma free colon cleanse, performed in a way that enhances rather than damages the electrical function of the cells, will take up to a year to complete. A colon cleanse can not be done safely, quickly. The risk of causing extreme irritation and subsequently increasing the risk of colon cancer is very real.

Herbal formulations that are combined using the knowledge of the electrical matrix of the individual herbs and their combined action is of paramount importance in any colon cleansing and rebuilding procedure. As a result of many, many years studying the electrical matrix of herbs, the industry leaders now have electrically correct herbal formulations (refer to Appendix).

Any herbal formulas created without an electrical understanding are mixtures that have the potential to cause more harm than good. Remember, as soon as you mix two of anything together, you change the electrical matrix and thus its behavior and thereby its interface with everything else.

Just because one herb has a diuretic effect and another a scouring action, putting the two together in the body may mean neither function takes place. This demonstrates the importance of knowing and understanding the electrical compatibility and the electrical function in anything we do to the body if we are to have any hope of cleaning up the mess humanity is currently in.

Every mouthful of food or drink that has ever passed between our lips, that was not taken in the right combination, not digested correctly, that contained any chemical substance, artificial sweetener or preservative, or did not contain nature's electrical construct, has an adverse impact on our colon and our general toxicity.

Chinese medicine believes every disease which manifests in the human body originates from imbalances within the colon. With our modern food manufacturing methods and serious overindulgence in sugar and wheat, there would be very few human beings in the western world who have healthy, nontoxic colons.

If you only took daily an electrically formulated herbal colon cleanse, you would be doing more to alleviate the toxic effects of modern living and eating than any other single thing you could possibly do. However, when combined with adequate levels of electrically correct hydration and at least thirty minutes a day of good physical lymphatic movement, you can exponentially decrease the future risk of disease manifestation and dramatically reduce any existing disease symptoms.

The cleaning of the body's lymphatic drainage system and lower digestive tract is of paramount importance in returning the body to homeostasis (electrical harmony) and achieving a long, disease-free life.

There is not one disease, not one malfunction that cannot be reversed. Your body desperately seeks its health and vitality. With a little bit of help on your behalf, it will respond beyond your wildest dreams.

Help us get this information out

You can do this by recommending your friends and family to purchase this book, or even buy extra copies and give it to them as presents. We can only continue to do the work and research by having sales of this book. Thank you for supporting us in this manner.

CHAPTER 12

LIFE - AN ELECTRICAL REALITY

In order for us to really feel at peace and in harmony we first have to find that harmony within. Once we find that harmony, it then acts as a ripple effect, rippling on out into our relationships, our families, our communities, our jobs. As everything in this universe is energy and all energy communicates with all other energy, it makes sense that if we focus on harmonizing our own reality first, then our energy will start radiating health and vitality, and attract to it similar energy.

In my last book, **Journey to Truth,** we discussed many of these energy concepts and suggested that a mastery of these perceptional realities gives us the keys to life, love, wealth and health. Everything is interrelated and connected.

We continue here in **Electrical Nutrition** to share specific, practical, self-help information. If you choose to implement this knowledge into your life, you will indeed benefit dramatically. Life will become more harmonious, love will bloom, wealth will start to flow and health - the starting point of it all - will continue to blossom into ever-increasing states of vitality and life-exuding bliss.

It could be said that there are a million causes of disease but in fact there is only one cause of disease and that is an electrical malfunction. However the electrical malfunction can be caused by a million different reasons. This is very obvious when we accept and understand the concept of an electrical universe. Without this acceptance we will always look in the wrong place for what we perceive are the answers to our problems.

From an electrical perspective, everything we do, feel and touch, and everything that everybody else does, has an impact on the frequencies of energy that are then released into this electrical universe of ours.

It is like a great soup bowl and every thought, word and deed, every ounce of pollution, every bit of everything, adds to the components of our soup bowl. We are not immune, any of us, from the effects of all these different frequencies, because our physicality, our emotions, our actions and our thoughts are all part of the ingredients of the soup.

Yet, within this gigantic mixture our consciousness, or the group of frequencies that condense into who we are, has an ability to govern which subtle frequencies impact on us. However, like a radio, we can only be receptive (conscious) to the frequencies that are being transmitted if we ourselves are tuned into that particular frequency. It is an electrical impossibility for a radio that is tuned to the AM band to pick up and play the song that is being transmitted by the FM station.

Our cellular structure, its behavior, function and health is totally governed by the frequency contained within it. Everything in this universe works with exactly the same laws which are sometimes referred to as natural law or cosmic law. However, a more accurate understanding would be to say that this universe works on the laws of energy.

It is even stated in the Bible that God is light, and the original word for light directly translates into the English word "energy." It is also said that God is everywhere. The one absolute, known by every scientific method, is that the only thing that is everywhere in this cosmos is "energy." In fact, the cosmos is energy.

Perhaps Jesus and many of the other great prophets were not talking about a religious reality but were in fact, within the confines of the vocabulary of the times, attempting to educate us about the construct of the universe so we could understand that we are a part of this great whole called God.

When we look at how energy manifests in this dimension, we find that the lower the frequency the more dense or solid is the physicality. It is this frequency change, to a lower vibratory rate, which manifests as increasing density in the cellular structure that is the start of all disease. As we load onto ourselves any disharmonic frequency, whether it be in the form of stress, physical impacts, chemical toxins, emotional reactivities, lifestyle choices, etc. we promote the densification of our cellular structure.

This electrical loading, as well as making every tissue in our body tighter, causes the electrical circuitry or the energy flow through our body's subtle electrical circuits, to be severely restricted. As the frequency drops, the flow is reduced, the cells compact in on themselves, our tissues become more dense, we tighten up, there is less blood flow, less lymphatic drainage, constricted bowels, tightening of the chest, constriction of the heart, etc., etc.

As all the physical restrictions take place, driven by a lowering of the frequencies contained in our energy fields, diseases in all their manifestations are the names and labels given to the way the physical body reacts to these constrictions of energy flow.

The symptoms that we rush off to our doctors or physiotherapists for, are all caused by this physical energetic reactivity. All malfunctions and disease states in the body can be traced energetically to the electrical malfunction and in fact can be diagnosed very simply by those able to be consciously aware of the subtle frequencies.

There are many therapists who, with little understanding of this energy communication, label it as psychic ability, medical intuitiveness and other so-called new age terminology. In fact, what is taking place is a very natural energy communication, something that is constantly happening between all aspects of this cosmos at all times.

It is not too difficult to learn to enhance our conscious awareness of this energy communication. Just as a radio can receive a transmission from a radio station if it is tuned into the same (right) frequency, so too can we tune into the frequency of what we are.

Likewise, most of the new age woo-woo and so-called special abilities and what some would term as spiritual gifts, are also these same perfectly natural, everyday energy communications. This conscious communication can be learned and mastered to an extremely high degree by anybody if they choose to get out of their ego and invest in the time to learn. It is not something that is a special gift any more than anybody who learns to do something very well.

We are energy and our energy is interfacing with all other energy at all times. We just have to become conscious of it.

There is not one part of our body that is not affected by everything we do and everything everybody else does. One of the most profound statements accredited to Jesus is, "Judge ye not." In fact, this is meant to be one of the cornerstones of Christianity.

Yet Jesus must have had a deep understanding of the energy interface between us all, because we are all affected by each other. There are times when we allow our behavior to be directly influenced by the frequency of energy that has been transmitted by somebody else.

This is an electrical universe. We are the highest life forms on this dimension and have an overbearing influence on the frequencies that surround and impact upon us. For example, if one of us allowed ourselves to get into our emotions and poured out our anger, that anger would be transmitted as a frequency of energy.

Three thousand miles away there may be somebody also experiencing their emotions who happened to be on that same frequency and zap!!! they take on the energy that was transmitted from us. Now they are really angry and their energy is sucking in any frequency that will add to their reality. Remember, birds of a feather flock together, or in modern language, energy is received on the same frequency that it was transmitted on.

The person three thousand miles away is now out of control and picking up more and more disharmonic frequencies from many different people until he explodes, picks up a gun and blows somebody away. Shock, horror, what a bad person, let's judge him, lock him up and throw the key away (and we think we are a Christian-based society). Remember Jesus and the "judge ye not?"

Perhaps the lesson for us here is that the person who exploded and blew somebody else away with a gun should be thanked by us because in fact, he just rephysicalized all the disharmonic frequencies that were transmitted by the rest of us. Yes, he may have pulled the trigger but who produced the frequencies of energy that were the disharmony he responded to? This is a closed electrical circuit. All frequency moves from physical to energy and then has to be rephysicalized - the circuit has to be completed.

Everything we transmit, every thought, word and deed is a frequency of energy that has to be rephysicalized.

This concept of rephysicalizing energy parallels the Christian saying of "what you sow, so shall you reap" and the Eastern laws of Karma. Perhaps the true message is that we have to look beyond our judgments to understand another reality, to embrace another consciousness, that of the electrical universe, because only then we will be able to see and understand that we are all one. Everything we do impacts upon each other, in fact, impacts on everything.

Everybody is looking for that magic pill, therapist, or the one technique they can use to cure all their aches, pains and illnesses (physical and emotional). There are very few who are actually committed to putting any investment of energy or time into their health and well-being. Almost everybody is looking for an answer outside of themselves.

It is time for people to take responsibility for themselves.

There is no reason why we should be unhealthy, in pain, or suffering in any way. Almost every dis-ease is reversible if you are willing to make that investment into yourself and a commitment to really becoming healthy. But you have to start with yourself! Remember? Thy Kingdom Come. We create the kingdom of heaven here, and "here" means in these bodies.

It was also said that the Kingdom of Heaven is guarded by the pearly gates. The only pearls (ivory) in our bodies are our teeth. Is this a metaphor that is telling us that our frequency, our health and our enlightenment is indexed to what comes in and what goes out of these pearly gates - our mouth?

Everything we take in through our mouth, and everything we expound (thought, word and deed) is a frequency of energy, and energy shapes everything - energy *is* everything.

We all control and create our own reality, everything around us, this earth, this consciousness and this universe. Our cells are the interface, our body is the temple that is the expression of God. For centuries we have lived and held our consciousness outside of our bodies. We have always been searching, desperately searching for our connection with all that is and it has been right here in front of us when we look in the mirror. Remember, Thy Kingdom Come. It is not out there somewhere, we are it.

It is fascinating to look at life's experiences (both good and bad) as gifts. And it is healthy to look at illness/accidents/ disease as gifts in disguise. They are often a wake-up call, a powerful message for us to open our eyes and see what we are doing to ourselves, to look at our habits, patterns and conditionings and reassess them. Are these beliefs really in my best interest? Am I really all that I can be or am I holding back in some way?

Certain physical states manifest in our bodies because we have been deaf to the subtle messages that have been reccurring over and over again. So the body finally realizes that you need a bigger hammer to make you see the woes of your ways. Louise Hay and Caroline Myss are two people who have brought to mainstream consciousness this viewpoint of looking beyond the physical to the other reasons behind illness.

It is important not to become too simplistic in our analysis and understand that each individual has his or her own unique set of circumstances and conditions surrounding their life situation. We should never put anyone in a box or assume that because they have, for example, developed stomach problems that it is automatically because they have undealt with emotional issues, or just because they have AIDS they have fallen into the victim mode or been sexually promiscuous, or just because we broke our foot it is because we are not walking our truth....

Sometimes "stuff happens!" Everyone has transmitted disharmonic frequencies and sometimes we are just rephysicalizing that disharmony if we happened to be tuned to that frequency at the time. Analysis often becomes our paralysis. It is much more advantageous to accept what has happened, learn from it and move on with our lives, focusing on what can help us enjoy life more fully and enable us to live a full and healthy life. Follow your bliss!

Remember we get a very good look at where we come from when we drive our car down the road backwards, but usually all hell will break out in front of us because we are not watching where we are going. Life is a forward path, a path that gives us experiences. We learn to accept these experiences by not taking them too seriously. It is only then that we can open up to the full joy, bliss and harmony that is our truth.

It is imperative that we challenge our own belief parameters about health and well-being. It is necessary to learn from our mistakes, not dwell on them and use them as excuses to get stuck in the bog, but rather accept them and move on. This cannot be emphasized enough. One of the keys to good health is: to look, to see, to understand, to accept and *to move on*.

In my many years of clinical experience, it has become obvious that it is possible to alleviate most conditions with advanced Vibrational Medical techniques, but inevitably people go back to their old ways and the original problem reoccurs. It is only possible to give people so much information, so much assistance (physically, emotionally and spiritually), but ultimately it is up to their willpower to actually take the bull by the horns and really make a difference.

That is why I do not like the term "healer." Nobody can heal anybody else. We can assist them in many ways. We can present them with a mirror so they can see themselves reflected therein. We can alleviate the stress loading on the cells. We can recharge the batteries, so to speak, and correct many of the electrical malfunctions. We can physically mend bones, sew up cuts, remove malfunctioning parts when there is no other option. We can explain nutrition and the importance of movement and how the body works. But what it really comes down to in the end is the person's determination to heal themselves. We cannot heal anybody else, we can only assist them on their own healing journey.

All of our life experiences are stored in our cellular memory as frequencies of energy. What we consciously remember could be described as only that which appears on the screen (of the computer), everything else is stored on the hard drive. It is all there. We may not be able to see it all at one time, but it is there.

It is possible to reduce the stress loading on our cellular structure by deleting some of the files that are no longer of any use, and we can also defrag the hard drive or simply stop adding so many files to our already-full memory.

It is important to add here that there are many different ways to clean up the hard drive (our cellular body). The long way is to pull up every old file, read through it and then throw it in the recycle bin. This is very laborious and time consuming, as well as being very tiring energetically. And often we go through this whole process and the old file ends up in the recycle bin and we forget that it actually still exists on our hard drive - that we have not completely removed it from our cellular memory, only regurgitated it and filed it in another part of the system.

This way of dealing with old files is very similar to many emotional release techniques and psychoanalytical practices in the Western world. Often a lot of time and energy is spent on bringing back up all the old files and going through them with a fine tooth comb. This is actually re-experiencing the scenarios again and reprogramming them onto the cellular structure once more without actually changing them in any way or deleting them at all, which was supposedly the aim of the process in the first place!

There are other ways to safely remove un-useful files from your cellular memory. Vibrational Medicine is a term based on the understanding that we consist of cells, which are made up of atoms, which are nothing except vibrating frequencies of energy.

If we and everything around us consist of vibrating frequencies of energy then it is easy to see that everything affects us in some way. Any "bad" or "negative" experience impacts upon our cellular structure as an electrical loading. These experiences could be seen as disharmonic frequencies of energy which lower the life force of the cells.

The aim of Vibrational Medicine is to encourage and facilitate participants to learn how to raise their vibrational frequency so that they can transmute any disharmonic frequency contained within their cellular structure.

In our schools we often use the image of a small smoldering campfire. We are often that small camp fire. If you can imagine somebody with a big wheel barrow full of wet leaves coming along and dumping them on our small campfire, the wet leaves would smother our small fire and snuff it out! And it really does feel like that sometimes. We struggle to keep our own fire burning and it certainly knocks us around when somebody comes along and dumps on us with either a lot of anger, or emotional outpouring of energy, or even when things just do not seem to be going right. If we are not in our power, if we are only a small smoldering campfire, these experiences will affect us dramatically.

The aim is not to get rid of the wet leaves in our lives - they exist and are a very important part of this whole experience. The objective is to build up our own fire and make it into a roaring bonfire so that those wet leaves no longer have a negative effect on us but rather can be used as fuel for our fire. The wet leaves dry up in our heat and then act as fuel! We can transmute what would initially be considered disharmonic energy into beneficial energy.

Similarly with our life experiences. We can chose to see them as "negative" and let them create disharmony in our lives, or transmute them in to a positive experience - learn from them and take those life experiences and use them to benefit ourselves. Understand that the gift of a heart attack may well be a total turn around of diet and lifestyle which may enable you to enjoy life much more and benefit greatly from this experience called life!

In order to transmute these so-called negative experiences into positive ones, we have to build our own fires first. We have to work on our own self-esteem, and fortify our own systems by supplementing our diets with electrically available nutrients, eating the right foods in the right combinations, being aware of the factors in our lives that create stress loading on our cellular structure, and ensuring that our body, heart and soul receives as much nourishment as possible, which would include joyful movement, lots of loving, and reflective quiet times.

As a participant at one of our schools in the United States said, "You have shown me that it is not a matter of getting rid of the darkness but rather turning on the light. You have helped me to find the switch."

Another one from a school in Canada said, "It's as if the ice is starting to melt and the sparks are starting to glow again..."

Sadly, there are many cases where, although the people were presented with all the information possible, they then chose not to continue on their path of growth and healing. Many times, I have been able to remove most of the stress loading from their system, re-energize their batteries and give them a taste of what it feels like to be in full health, but they return to their old ways.

One could use the analogy of a truck laden with rocks struggling up a steep hill. We are that truck, life is that steep incline, and the rocks are our accumulation of stress and experiences that weigh us down. The truck can only take so much and there are only a limited number of repairs that can be done until it can no longer do the job it was designed to do.

We are the same. Our bodies can only take so much. There are only so many pills we can take to suppress the pain, which is a symptom of an electrical malfunction. If we do not address the causes of the malfunction and take some of the loading off, we too will soon stop working completely. To return to full health we have to reduce the load. Sometimes this requires us to make some very difficult lifestyle choices, but that is the experience, the joy of living, learning to make these choices.

To be healthy and happy is a full-time occupation. It does not have to be a laborious, difficult or painful process. It can be fun and can be integrated into your present lifestyle. It is more a conscious choice we can all make to be more aware about what we put into our bodies, how our bodies react, how we feel in certain situations, and what our needs truly are - what is it that gives us joy, that makes us feel happy and healthy?

Health and happiness is not found in a pill or in a doctor's consultation room. True health and happiness is a learned process, the key is inside you. The way to find it is to have determination and the will to invest your time and energy into yourself. And remember, follow your bliss. Make each moment a joyful one, each mouthful of food a nourishing one, each experience a chance to learn something new, and each connection with another an opportunity to share love, to be love and to experience this experience called life without limits, to love without limits, to be without limits.

But remember, we cannot share that which we do not have, so start with loving and accepting yourself. Look after these bodies, they are our only vehicle of experience this time around. Electrical nutrition is the key to electrical harmony. Electrical harmony is the key to your bliss, health, wealth and enlightenment... And do not forget, seriousness is outlawed... Enjoy!

In Light and Love, ***Denie and Shelley.***

Help us get this information out

You can do this by recommending your friends and family to purchase this book, or even buy extra copies and give it to them as presents. We can only continue to do the work and research by having sales of this book. Thank you for supporting us in this manner.

RESOURCES, REFERENCES & RECOMMENDED BOOKS

The Milk Book – How Science is Destroying Nature's Nearly Perfect Food by William Campbell Douglas, M.D. A must read for anyone who wants the truth about dairy products. One of the most complete pieces of scientific information written on the human interface with dairy products and we respectfully suggest that nobody should ever comment about dairy food products until they have read this book. Available through 1 800 728 2288 / 770 399 5617.

Beyond Probiotics by Ann Louise Gittleman, M.S., C.N.S., author of 40/30/30 Phenomenon. Discusses the importance of a healthy biological terrain and the lack of healthy soil. A Keats Good Health Guide, for more information call 800 622 8986, or email: defensecom@earthlink.net

Shots in the Dark by Barbara Loe Fisher. On the devastation of mass vaccinations. Email: BarbaraLoeFisher@nextcity.com

The Virus and the Vaccine Atlantic Monthly, Feb. 2000. Visit: www.feat.org for more info.

Unraveling the Mystery of Autism and Pervasive Developmental Disorder: A Mother's Story of Research and Recovery by Karyn Seroussi & Bernard Rimland, PhD. Tying Autism in with vaccinations. Available through Amazon.com

Scientific Investigation into Chinese Qigong by Richard H. Lee, China Healthways Institute, 115 N. El Camino Real, San Clemente, CA 92672, Call 1 800 743 5608.

Thyroid Inhibiters by Lita Lee, Ph.D., To Your Health Newsletter, Vol. 5, No. 1, Jan. 2000, email: litaleephd@aolc.om. Discusses importance of animal protein and devastation of Soy, raw broccoli, and unsaturated oils.

Nourishing Traditions by Sally Fallon. The cookbook that challenges politically correct nutrition and diet dictocrats. (1999, 2nd Edition New Trends Publishing - 1 877 707 1776 or 219 268 2601) www.westonaprice.org

Know Your Fats by Mary G. Enig, PhD. The Complete Primer for understanding the nutrition of fats, oils and cholesterol. (2000, Bethesda Press) www.bethesdapress.com

The Politics of Cancer Revisited by Dr. Samuel Epstein.

Questioning Chemotherapy by Ralph W. Moss, M.D.

Thermotherapy a new treatment that encourages the natural healing of hemorrhoids. Contact: Roger Estes, 1526 S. Ash, Spokane, WA 99203, tel: 509 456 6090, fax: 509 624 3140

Virtual Daylight - Clear Vision, Contact: Alan Henderson, PO Box 1865, Wellington, New Zealand, tel: +64 4 499 0012, fax: +64 4 499 0014, email: hengrp@voyager.co.nz, website: www.virtualdaylight.com. The latest advances on healthy lighting in the workplace.

Clean Energy Combustion Systems provide State of the Art Combustion Technology with Higher Efficiencies, Cleaner Emissions, and Lower Costs. Contact: John Thuot, 7087 MacPherson Ave., Burnaby, BC V5J 4N4, Canada, tel: 604 435 9339, Fax: 604 435 9329, website: www.cecsi.com

Let them eat dirt an article by Michael Downey, in the Toronto Star, 10 Jan. 1999.

APPENDIX

The information contained in this appendix is based on the honestly held beliefs of the authors pertaining to the integrity and performance of the products and information known at the time of writing. No guarantees, endorsements or levels of response are given or implied. No products or services are specifically recommended other than as reflections of our experience based on personal usage and clinical experience of over fifteen years. These products and/or services have distinguished themselves, but in no way do we feel this is a full and complete list. This list consists of those that have come to our attention at this time. It is not our intention to discredit any company's products by their omission.

The impetus to produce this publication has been motivated by the strong desire to give people the information that there are some extraordinarily effective products on the market today. These products can assist the body in its detoxification process, which is the single biggest requirement to reverse the degeneration process that is rampant in the western world. Our other motivating factor was to make apparent the misinformation that has become the mindset of many in the Western world regarding what is desirable nutrition and what is a healthy diet. To that end the following list of products on the next pages is supplied which have been sourced throughout the world.

Electrically Available Natural Nutritional Supplements
Available through Avena Originals Health Club

A friendly, small, family-owned herb company. On the advice of Denie Hiestand, along with their own line of herbal supplements, they are now stocking a high quality range of electrically formulated, electrically available herbs and supplements so that you can get everything from the one place.

U.S.A./Canada Orders/info 1 800 207 2239
From Overseas 403 314 2351
Fax line **U.S.A./Canada** 1 888 352 5145
Fax line from Overseas 403 314 2081
email:avena@telusplanet.net   **www**.avenaoriginals.com

Note:- **These products are made from the highest grade pure natural Herbs and Oils. They are not drugs that act quickly to suppress physical problems, they are foods that are electrically combined that nourish and rebuild the body on a daily basis over time.**
It is important to understand it is not the individual ingredients that are the active agents, but rather the electrical combination and its subsequent interaction, as a whole, with the body's system.

NEWSFLASH!   NEWSFLASH!

Electrical Nutrition™ Professional is a line of electrically available,™ electrically forumlated,™ natural nutritional supplements containing nature's electrical matrix.™ This is an exclusive line for health professionals only. If you are a health professional who would like to make this line available to your clients contact us below, or if you would like your health professional to carry these electrically formulated health products tell them to contact us.

Telephone: 425 785 3468
Fax: 917 464 8128
Email: info@vibrationalmedicine.com

The following is a list of products available from Avena Originals Health Club.

CLEANSING:

Herb Cocktail – an electrically formulated combination of Hibiscus, Psyllium husk, Peppermint, Licorice, Cascara Sagrada, Siberian Ginseng, Corn Silk. The final ingredient to make this combination electrically available is to mix the powder with about a half a glass of pure unsweetened orange juice before ingesting. The easiest way to mix this is in a small bottle or container with a lid, and shake vigorously. Herb Cocktail is a gentle, yet thorough cleanse to be taken daily over a six-month to one-year period. Amounts vary per person. For children, a quarter of a teaspoon first thing each morning is usually sufficient. For adults, it can range between half to one teaspoon once or twice daily, depending on the level of detoxification desired. It is best to take Herb Cocktail on an empty stomach, first thing in the morning or last thing at night. It really helps create soft, regular bowel movements and, by cleaning out the "gunk," people usually experience enhanced energy levels.

H/C Plus – is encapsulated for convenience which means it is not as powerful as Herb Cocktail. It combines electrically Psyllium, Licorice, Cascara Sagrada, Red Clover, Kelp. Sometimes H/C Plus is better for women with very sensitive systems or for those who find mixing the Herb Cocktail powder with orange juice too difficult. Normal dose rate is four to eight capsules once daily, to be taken with live water.

Para Cleanse – an encapsulated electrically available combination of Psyllium, Licorice, Dulse, Red Raspberry, Black Walnut, Cascara Sagrada, Red Clover, Cat's Claw. Designed specifically as a parasite cleanse. Take three to four capsules once or twice daily with pure, live water.

REBUILDING:

N-Zymes – an electrically formulated combination of seven active enzymes: Protease, Amylase, Cellulase, Maltase, Lactase, Phytase, Sucrase, to aid digestion. Taken with meals, two to four per meal is recommended or more if needed. These are the building blocks of our body – the workers, without them we cannot exist very happily.

Friendly Flora – consists of two live organisms: L. Salivarius, L. Plantarium that are electrically compatible. These are two of the necessary Flora that we need to help digestion and to fight candida. Especially good for those who have had antibiotic treatments. Take one to two capsules daily (or more if needed) on an empty stomach with pure, live water.

Flora Balance-The B.O.D. Strain of Bifidus - Comes in 3 names: Latero-Flora from your health professional, Flora Balance from Avena Health Club, and Supreme Flora from the health food store (if you can find one that carries it). Harvested from beneath the ice tundra, it has not been mutated by atmospheric nuclear testing so is the ultimate Candida fighter. A must for any Candida program or to rebuild the gut bacteria after antibiotics. Recommended for Candida control: 20-30 capsules a day for three days, then reduce to 4 capsules a day for the rest of the month. Then repeat saturation (20-30 a day for 3 days), then 2 a day for at least 3 months.

Minerals – Real at Last – a unique combination of electrically compatible proportions of Potassium, Magnesium, Calcium, Iron, Zinc, Manganese, Copper, Chromium, Selenium, Molybdenum, Vanadium from electrically available sources. We need to supplement our mineral intake due to modern food processing and handling which often depletes our food of the necessary minerals. Take one to two capsules daily with food.

STRENGTHENING:

Electric C – is one of the most powerful immune boosters known to exist. It consists of electrically available Vitamin C, Potassium, Sodium, Magnesium, Zinc. All the important electrolyte salts. This powder, when mixed with half a glass of pure, unsweetened orange juice or milk, is electrically synergetic with our bodies. Mix thoroughly (by vigorous shaking) in a small bottle or container with a lid on and then drink straight away. To be taken on a daily basis to ward off colds and flu, to help the body cope with environmental pollution, also great for smokers to help reduce toxic build-up. Take in larger quantities, three to four times a day, if fighting a cold or other more serious conditions.

Toco – is an electrical blend of Tocopherols and Tocotrienols which are powerful natural antioxidants. Contains amino acids and phytonutrients to help maintain optimum health and provide control of free radicals within the body. Especially good before and after athletic activity, times of high work stress and extremely beneficial for post-operative recovery. Often used as a cholesterol reducer and to assist in balancing a vegetarian diet. The total "B" group supplemention.

Rejuvenate – contains Capsicum, Cayenne, Siberian Ginseng, Zinc, Potassium, Gingko Biloba, Licorice in an electrically compatible combination. It helps to fire up the system and get the energy moving. Take two to four capsules per day with pure, live water and food.

Herbal Plus – another electrically formulated combination of Gingko Biloba Licorice, Capsicum, Eleuthrococcus Senticosis especially good for activating the brain cells before studying, athletic performance, or if you work a lot with computers. Clears the head! Take two to four capsules with a full glass of pure, live water.

Herbal Eze – contains Black Cohosh, Bayberry, Cat's Claw, Wood Betany, Capsicum, Uva Ursi, Parsley, Red Raspberry. This electrical combination can assist those with hormonal imbalances, PMS, period problems. Take three to four capsules with a full glass of pure, live water, once a day or as required.

H2O Plus – electrically suspended particles of silver that can dramatically assist with repetitive ear aches (put two drops in the ear morning and night) and acts as a natural antibiotic (taken orally, but do not swallow). Because of its antibiotic qualities it is not advisable to ingest as this will have the effect of killing the active bacteria, enzymes and flora. Allow the liquid to stay in the mouth for as long as possible so it can electrically interface through the saliva, then spit it out. You can also gargle with it as often as required.

Colostrum - Avena is now stocking New Life Colostrum which is the world's best naturally produced, low heat processed Colostrum from New Zealand pasture fed cows. Mix two teaspoons of powder into quarter-half a glass of water, shake vigorously in a small bottle. Add maple syrup to taste if required. For a very powerful breakfast drink for those on the go, add a raw free-range fertilized egg to the above mixture and shake well. It tastes really good! You will also be amazed at what it will do for your libido!!!

Notes to Colostrum

Colostrum is the pre-milk fluid produced from the mammary glands during the first 72 hours after birth. It builds up the immune system of a newly born. The cow produces far more Colostrum than is needed by its calf. Quite often much of the Colostrum was discarded as there was too much produced. Now the industry has discovered a wonderful use of this overabundance of Colostrum. Many human babies do not receive any mother's Colostrum at all, and if you were ever vaccinated, immunized or given antibiotics, the effects of that Colostrum would have been almost voided. We have sourced the best Colostrum in the world and now make it available through Avena's 1 800 number. We will also have this Colostrum as part of our Electrical Nutrition Professional line.

New Zealand has the most pure, most effective, most potent Colostrum in the world. All of New Zealand's Colostrum is marketed by a company that calls it New Life Colostrum. Their Colostrum is collected only from New Zealand pasture-fed cows which are free from pesticides, antibiotics and hormones. The New Zealand Dairy Group has spent millions of dollars to perfect the processing of Colostrum so that its potency and effectiveness remains at the highest level possible. We have personally met the scientist that developed this technology and also the owner of the company that markets New Life Colostrum in North America. Both were very integruous and they certainly have put their heart and soul into this product.

What makes this Colostrum so unique is that it comes from pasture-fed cows. When cows are pasture-fed it means they are exposed to a much larger number of natural pathogens than in a feedlot, and therefore, their Colostrum is much more potent in transferring immunity to these pathogens to humans. Plus, when a cow eats green grass instead of dried, processed feed, it is getting all the natural nutrients and live enzymes it is designed to get. This live, raw food means the animal's Colostrum is much more potent and effective. In other words, it is more electrically available and contains nature's electrical matrix.

Colostrum helps support the immune system, it helps enhance skin and muscle rejuvenation, build lean muscle mass, and maintain a healthy intestinal flora.

NOURISHING THE SKIN

Precious Oils for the Face – a special combination of electrically compatible essential oils that soak into the pores of the skin. The electrical availability is noticeable because it leaves no oily residue – it is completely absorbed and utilized as food for the skin. Totally natural and made with the purest essential oils. Use sparingly.

Body Splash – electrically combined oils of Almonds, Orange, Lime. Great for the whole body. Nourishes the skin, protects it, softens it. Good to use before and after swimming, lying in the sun, on the hands if you work with chemicals, and on dry areas of the body.

Tooth Oil – electrically available combination of oils that stimulate the gums, and clean the teeth without the harsh abrasives and sugar content normally found in commercial toothpastes. Put four drops on your toothbrush and brush normally. You can swallow it and this acts as a stomach calmer, and mouth freshener. Smaller amounts can be used by children. After the initial surprise at the intensity of this powerful electrical combination, children and adults grow to love the fresh taste.

Foot Oils – combine the essential oils of Eucalyptus, Peppermint, Camphor to create a soothing electrical formulation for tired and sore feet. Stimulates the reflex points on the feet also.

Massage Oil – an electrical combination of Almond, Peppermint, Wintergreen, Eucalyptus, Camphor. Use sparingly on sore muscles. Can be used before and after athletic activity. Keep well away from the eyes or other sensitive areas.

Electrically Tuned Rebounders - tuned to the body's electromagnetic frequency, these rebounders have been created with the understanding that we are electrical, that all energy connects with all other energy, is affected by and affects all other energy. This is one of the best pieces of health equipment for use by the whole family to facilitate adequate lymphatic drainage (imported to North America by Avena Originals). The world's only Electrically Tuned Rebounder.

Bounce Back Fitness Chair - Lymphatic drainage for those who are not able to use the electrically tuned rebounder. Available through Avena at 1 800 207 2239.

Q-Link - helps reduce the negative effects of EMF (electromagnetic fields) from cell phones, computers, commercial air travel etc. Q-Links contains an embedded chip and micro-circuit that acts like a tuning fork, rebalancing you. Assists in keeping you relaxed, present, centered. The Q-Link comes as a pendant to hang around your neck under your cloths. There are many EMF blockers on the market but the Q-Link has more science and electrical research data. It is also personally recommended and used by Denie & Shelley Hiestand. Now available by calling Avena at 1 800 207 2239.

Microhydrin

To order contact Alia Aurami at:
Phone .... 1 877 ALIVE 00 (1-877-254-8300)
From Overseas call 425 785 3468
email:alia@gnaccess.com
Or order direct from the web by visiting
www.rbcglobenet.com/vibrationalmedicine.asp

Microhydrin - Combines a miniscule silica atom with hydrogen modified to carry an extra electron. The loosely bound extra electron, which has been attached to the hydrogen, is easily given up to neutralize harmful free radicals. Its unique chemical structure literally pulls oxygen from the bloodstream into the cells. Most antioxidants such as Vitamin C, Vitamin E, Beta-carotene, Selenium, and OPCs from grape seed or pine bark consist of large complex molecules that donate one of their electrons which then attaches itself to a free radical, thus neutralizing it. But, once it loses its electron, it then becomes a free radical itself. Dr. Patrick Flanagan overcame this effect by discovering a way to attach an extra electron to the hydrogen enhanced silicate mineral so that it can freely give an electron yet not become a free radical itself in the process. Taking Microhydrin can help combat the harmful effects of pollution and stress, help increase mental clarity and energy, help with bacterial or viral infections, respiratory and circulatory conditions, insect bites and stings, is beneficial for smokers or people exposed to second-hand smoke, can enhance athletic performance, amongst other benefits. We use it primarily to lower the surface tension of the water we drink so that it can hydrate our cells more effectively. Please note, if you take prescription medicines or insulin please ask your physician to monitor you and adjust your dosages where appropriate. **To make water electrically alive,** empty one capsule into a liter of drinking water. DO NOT use a plastic water container. Use glass.

Also available from the same source as Microhydrin is:
Spirulina - microclustered, organic protein and amino acid supplement.

Supreme Flora Yogurt

Karikaas Natural Dairy Products Ltd.,
156 White Rock Road, R.D. 2, Rangiora, New Zealand.
email: info@karikaas.co.nz   **www.**karikaas.co.nz
Phone 03 312 8708
Fax 03 312 8208
Supreme Yogurt (containing the B.O.D. strain of Bifidus, a world first and only licensed manufacturer). Great for fighting Candida or to rebuild gut bacteria after antibiotic usage. **Possibly the best natural Yogurt in the world.** Karikaas, makers of quality dairy products and European cheeses.
Supreme Flora (the B.O.D. strain) capsules are available from Karikaas if you cannot get the yogurt in your area of New Zealand.
The yogurt is sadly not available in North America but the capsules of B.O.D. strain are available from the Avena Health Club (see Pg. 190).

Electrically Available Meal Ideas

A general outline of some suggestions of what to eat and when. Outlined are food combinations that are electrically available to the body, that the body recognizes as nutrition and can digest a lot easier. It is not that difficult to change the patterns and you will feel so much lighter and have more energy for your busy lives. And your body will thank you for it! One side effect of eating electrically combined food groups is that you will notice the toxic waste dump (cellulite and bulging bellies) will significantly reduce. Helped by taking an electrically-formulated Herbal Cleanse in the morning and electrically available enzymes with each big meal. The main thing is to enjoy eating, appreciate the food, put lots of loving energy into preparing it and do not be too hard on yourself if you have a craving for something not electrically available - just take some extra Avena enzymes!

BREAKFAST:
Start with a banana and take a couple of other pieces of fruit to eat throughout the morning. Drink lots of live, electrically available water all day.

LUNCH:
Option 1. A protein salad - such as green lettuce with boiled eggs, bacon bits, avocado, raw vegetables like carrots sliced thinly, tomatoes, with a balsamic vinegar and olive oil dressing.

Option 2. A carbohydrate salad - such as a potato salad or one made with sweet potatoes, use a light mayonnaise (or vinaigrette), red onions or spring onions to spice it up, plus salt and pepper.

Option 3. Grapes and Dutch Gouda cheese or other good cheese with no food coloring and/or half an avocado with salt and pepper, balsamic vinegar and olive oil.

Option 4. Baked Potato with a little butter, or refried potato - Swiss Style (hash browns / Rosti), and salad.

Option 5. A free range organic / fertile egg omelette with mushrooms, onions, tomatoes, cheese, cream cheese and salmon (some or all of the combinations), with a little green salad.

Option 6. Sausages, bacon and eggs with a raw tomato and onion salad, or fried mushrooms, onions and garlic.

Option 7. A hearty vegetable soup, chicken and vegetable soup, or meat and vegetable soup.

DINNER:

If you had a carbohydrate lunch then have some protein for dinner or vice versa.

Option 1. Fresh Pacific Salmon cooked in butter, with steamed or lightly stir-fried vegetables (no potatoes or corn).

Option 2. Tenderloin Steak (or other good quality beef) cut into strips and lightly stir-fried with onions, garlic and fresh vegetables.

Option 3. Steak with steamed broccoli and a raw tomato and onion salad with a balsamic / olive oil dressing.

Option 4. A potato dinner with vegetables. Can also use sweet potato and pumpkin.

    a) baked potatoes,

    b) pan-fried potatoes, or

    c) a potato casserole baked in the oven with butter and onions (boil potatoes beforehand and fry onions in a little butter then place in layers).

Option 5. Chickpea or bean casserole with vegetables. Can place a layer of cheese on top and grill it to make it crusty and brown before serving.

Option 6. Free-range cooked chicken, roasted, cold, or baked in a casserole, with vegetables.

Option 7. Slow roasted leg of lamb with pumpkin and onions cooked with it. Serve with carrots and peas and a fresh mint sauce (chop mint finely and mix with vinegar).

Simple, easy, no fuss meals. Fresh, healthy and visually appealing. Bon appetite!

PLEASE NOTE:

The absolute "no-no" foods are:
Artificial sweetener, pop, margarine, foods with any chemicals, artificial flavors, enhancers, additives, preservatives, colorings or any food that has been changed from the way nature made it.
Foods that should be eaten in extreme moderation are:
Sugar, all grains, which includes bread, pasta, donuts, burger buns, pizza, muffins, breakfast cereal - in other words, anything made with wheat and/or other grains.

The best food is:
Everything nature has made, in the way nature made it, in other words, all fresh fruit, all fresh vegetables, potatoes, pumpkin, squash, sweet potato, yams, etc., alive unsweetened and uncolored dairy products (natural butter, cheese, yogurt), top quality meat, fish, wild game, free range fertile eggs and chickens and all other organic animal and vegetable produce.
The only question you have to ask yourself before eating is:
Did nature make this the way I am about to eat it?
If the answer is "Yes," eat it, and if the answer is "No," it could be more "toxin" than "nutrition."

Keep it fresh, keep it raw, keep it high vibration, keep the proteins and carbohydrates separate, keep it simple and enjoy!

International Academy of Vibrational Medical Science
info. on next page.

INTERNATIONAL ACADEMY of
VIBRATIONAL MEDICAL SCIENCE

Canada   New Zealand   Switzerland   U.S.A.

100 Warren Street, Suite 1402
Jersey City, NJ U.S.A.   07302

Ph. 425 785 3468
Fax 917 464 8128

E-mail: info@vibrationalmedicine.com
www.vibrationalmedicine.com

The International Academy of Vibrational Medical Science offers experiential in-depth learning intensives at the highest level. These advanced courses include the full spectrum of leading edge discoveries in Vibrational Medicine, Energy Awareness, Emotional/ Mental Mastership, Sexuality, Personal Relationships, Movement & Music, Kinesiology, Nutritional Training and Energy Mastership. The Academy's courses are taught around the world.

Contact the Academy at the above address or e-mail to:
info@vibrationalmedicine.com

Visit the Academy's web site at:
www.vibrationalmedicine.com

International Academy of Vibrational Medical Science

*An integrated school of awareness to
rapidly expand your consciousness.*

Statement of Intent:

Dear Seekers,

*We are excited to have created a world class
school of learning that will assist you in your path of
awareness, so you may grow spiritually and
emotionally to achieve everything that you are.*

*The purpose of the school is to assist you in
attaining your own healing and self-mastery, so you
can become that totally powerful, loving and free
being that you are, and with that help humanity.*

*At the same time, you will be introduced to one
of the most advanced methods of healing currently
available on the planet, that of Vibrational Medicine.*

*This will take your knowledge from a basic
understanding of the body's electromagnetic energy
circuits, to your connection with the unseen world
beyond, and culminating, if you so desire, with total
mastery of your emotions and releasing all your
limitations.*

*These intensives (trainings) are very powerful
gatherings which seek the unfolding of the highest in
each of us. The message is clear: "The Time is Now" to
fully understand, realize and live the truth of who you
are, without fear, dogma or restriction of your
expression in any way.*

Each intensive will be unique because people come with their own unique desires and levels of willingness to learn, stretch, and go beyond.

The entire focus of the Academy's teachings will be for you to find and express your own Empowerment, Freedom and Truth. You will be introduced to beliefs and understandings from many cultures and societies, ancient and modern, from this earth and beyond, so you can develop your own perceptions, realities and truths.

These trainings are very powerful, life changing, heart opening experiences. This is the Mastership School and has profound effects on all who avail themselves of it.

"Everything is energy. Energy is everything. Once you learn to master energy, you can be the master of everything: Life, Love, Wealth and Health."

Denie Hiestand.

Thus the objectives of the International Academy of Vibrational Medical Science are:

◆   To bring participants to a point of consciousness that will allow them to know and experience their fullest expression of the power, gloriousness and greatness they are.

◆   To bring participants to a point of consciousness that allows them to be free of any dogma, limiting belief structures or inhibitions.

◆   To show women that they are allowed, and in fact, should and can, take back their power and self-worth and that they have a right to be all that they are, including being powerful and free.

◆   To show men that they can honor their maleness, and, at the same time, let go their ego-based domination, control and emotional reactivity. To show them that they can open their hearts, learn to feel, to unconditionally love, to increase their power and self-worth with full expression and honor.

◆   To bring participants to a point of consciousness so that they can live this life without any limitations (mentally, physically and expressively) and in a state of total joy, bliss and honor. "I am free, free to be, totally me."

◆   To create an awareness and a comprehensive understanding of how to maintain their own and/or their family/ clients' health and happiness by using their knowledge of the body's electrical system with a full understanding of Vibrational Medical Science.

A further objective for those who desire to continue their training in the Vibrational Medical Science Practitioner Program, is to ensure participants are highly trained, fully informed, capable and professional practitioners of Vibrational Medicine - the Health Care of the future.

Or to enter the Personal Growth Program to pursue their further development in personal growth, tantra, sexuality, relationships, personal freedoms and expression, to fully live life without limits.

The International Academy of Vibrational Medical Science, so you can be,
                          "Free to Be, Totally Me."

The Academy offers the following course of studies:

Vibrational Medical Science Practitioner Program.
Personal Growth Program.
Master Practitioner Certificate Program.
Vibrational Medical Science Degree Program.

The following is a brief outline of two of the Academy's many courses:

VB001: Energy Awareness
(5 day - 40 hour intensive)

This course focuses on understanding energy, energy patterns, flows and meridians. The emphasis is on physicalizing the energy, experiencing it and raising your vibrational frequencies through awareness, music and movement. Gain greater awareness of yourself in relation to the whole. Learn to honor yourself and each other. Move away from judgments of yourself and others. Become aware of the energy frequencies that allow past traumas to be held onto.

This course will also start the process that takes you to a new frequency, that of the heart, to remove and transmute all disharmonic frequencies. You will start the learned process of enlightenment. An introduction to some meditation techniques will help center yourself, aid the discovery of your purpose/direction, and enhance the development of self-acceptance and honor. Nature trips are included to heighten your awareness of energy.

The focus is always on increasing your conscious awareness of Energy. This course has the potential to be the most life changing week you will ever experience. Powerful, dynamic and full on, this is the Mastership school.

Suggested reading, "Journey to Truth" by Denie Hiestand.

VB002: Emotional Mental Mastership (8 day - 80 hour intensive - prerequisite VB001)

This course will assist in awakening the Body, Heart and Soul to their full potential. You will become aware of the ninety percent of yourself that has no conscious reality. You will dive within, take the plunge, face your fears and overcome them. You will free yourself from the shadows of the past by releasing parental and societal patterns.

You will learn to change the frequency of your cells to detraumatize your body, free your mind and release your soul. You will release the chains and blockages in your chakras and allow your creative, expressive, energy to flow in all areas without limits.

This mastership is attained by using that extra part of yourself that you will rediscover. You are complete in every way. By increasing your vibratory rate that completeness becomes your reality.

Become one with yourself and everything around you through the experience of your soul merge. Expand your consciousness so you can live free of any limitations. Learn to truly hear the voices from deep within which are your conscious connections with your higher self (frequencies).

These eight days will be spent looking within and being honest, freeing yourself from your emotions, your blockages, your dogmas and belief structures. Finding and living this newfound part of yourself, you will experience your greatness, your love, your passion, your joy, bliss and honor.

Contact the Academy for further information.

Testimonials
Next page.

Testimonials for the IAVMS

"In my recent spiritual work, I encountered a quote: "A psychologist only mends you, he doesn't transform you." As a psychologist, I found this to be all too true. Thus, with great delight, I have encountered Denie Hiestand and his transformational work. The courses offered by the International Academy of Vibrational Science are a must take for those who seek to transform themselves."

Dr. Stephen Vizzard, PhD. Seattle, WA. U.S.A.

"I have learnt more attending the IAVMS schools than I did in all my time at medical school."

Dr. Mary Pellicer, MD.Yakima, WA. U.S.A.

"As a medical doctor and student of Denie's International Academy of Vibrational Medical Science, the Christ force healing energy Denie teaches us to open our hearts to, is truly one of the most extraordinary, powerful, profound experiences of my entire life."

Dr. Linda C. Hole, MD. Spokane, WA. U.S.A.

"Attention, all you mid-life crisis-ing baby booming, health professionals. . . this man can truly lead you into a more satisfying and meaningful life as a healer. I know."

Dr. Frederick Kimball, MD. Everett, WA. U.S.A.

"I would not hesitate to send any of my clients to your training. Each of you model what self acceptance is. You really gave me food for thought about "self esteem" and "intention," terms bandied about so much among therapy groupies. Your training is very practical and yet jumps to the esoteric so easily. Because of your insistence upon simple function, subjects like kundalini become safe and possible."

Dr. Roger Ehlert, PhD. Coeur d'Alene, Idaho. U.S.A.

"In reality it is a question of consciousness, a slow process to which Denie and Shelley provide stimulus with public presentations, but mostly with lively and invigorating courses and workshops. They provide food for the body, mind and soul."

Peter Baumann, PhD. Basel. Switzerland.

"Every Health Care Professional should do this course! I have just completed my Chinese Medicine Degree and this course was the icing on the cake."

Louis Fassbind, CM. Rigi-Staffel. Switzerland.

"Something has shifted in me. I'm 24 years old and I've been living in fear of always doing the right thing - it's time for me to listen to my heart and do my thing."

Deborah, Nelson, B.C. Canada.

"Denie got to me and I opened up and felt energy from plants, trees, rocks and people, saw their auras and much more. I arrived home a new, loving person, resonating on a higher frequency, glowing with total awareness to everything. He has taught me to be a Master of my Being."

Ester, Invercargill. New Zealand.

"Finally spirituality and science in one. I honor Denie for his integrity, mastery and courage to walk that fine line of the leading edge. I am grateful to have found my connection with my heart. I can now make a real difference. Thank you Denie and Shelley for the blessing you have been to me. Your book, Journey to Truth really propelled me to do the (IAVMS) courses and the incredible electrical private work on me are the reasons I now can say I came back to life and have simple, grounded tools for raising my vibration and becoming more of who I am. I feel peace, joy and feel more present and in my essence...."

Afra, Victoria, B.C. Canada.

""I feel Oprah should devote an entire show to Denie and Shelley Hiestand's program "Energy Awareness." Denie was an electrical engineer, then a dairy farmer, and now a most gifted healer. During his life he has kept his eyes and heart wide open to every experience and has combined his knowledge of science (electricity, nutrition) to understand the powerful laws of the universe. His head fought this calling for years but his heart finally won out.

Shelley is a dancer with an intuitive and profound understanding of global music and its affect on our energy centers or chakras and cells. She embodies, and shows us how to embody, increased vibrational frequencies so that we may evolve faster and enjoy life more fully and completely.

Combined, Denie and Shelley have the most profound program which combines Denie's knowledge of the electrical nature of the universe (science) with its physical and spiritual implications for us. All of this knowledge and wisdom comes at a time when the planets are aligning, the electrical forces in our universe are polarizing and we have the best opportunity to evolve faster and higher than ever before.

Before attending this course, I knew much of this information. Hearing it again from Denie reconfirmed everything I had learned. But that was all in my head. The power of this course is that it connects the head with the spirit and with the body. Shelley's dance and movement brings the natural laws of the universe into our bodies and changes us forever. It is the complete package.

During the course, I was able to FEEL the wisdom and knowledge of the universe and become one with it. Since taking the course, my own work has been far more powerful, I find people on the street are drawn to me with twinkling eyes, and at 45 I have more energy and stamina than my teenage children! I approach life with confidence and assurance. Problems become insignificant. Joy is everywhere.

I was a tough sell. I am skeptical of gurus and followers. I am a well educated educator and business person who reads voraciously. I do not waste my time on things that do not matter."

Leslie, Victoria, B.C. Canada.

"I have been a teacher of Transcendental Meditation for 25 years, a Reiki Master, Nutritional Consultant and Massage Therapist. I have also experienced over 700 of a variety of "healing" sessions. I unquestionably rate the Academy's first and second levels as the two most valuable things to be done by any person seeking expanded self awareness and greater happiness in daily life. Rather than addressing individual problems (darkness) and trying to figure out how to get rid of the darkness, Denie and Shelley show you how to simply turn on the light."

Allen Glonek, Fairfield, Iowa. U.S.A.

"In twenty-five years of searching, including trips to India, this course has made it possible for me to move further, faster and safer along my path than anything I have previously experienced. The International Academy of Vibrational Medical Science course as taught/channelled by Denie Hiestand is one, if not the most powerful tool that any of us can avail ourselves with to propel us towards enlightenment."

Elizabeth, Caenarfon. Wales.

"I have done several seminars including the Barbara Brennan School of Healing and this course (IAVMS) has been the most beneficial to me to date. I found the size of the group provided me with a much safer feeling which helped me to show up more. I was also very impressed with the amount of love and honor which I felt. I would highly recommend this course to anyone who has any interest what so ever - you will not be disappointed."

Jennifer, Seattle. U.S.A.

"Whoo! Quite some week. It has been fabulous to take some more time with myself and be inside and see the change within. The peace I've gained is incredible. Shelley, you are an amazing person. I enjoyed your love, laughter and light. Denie, you are the blessing I've been waiting for. My legs feel great and the cells are having a ball."

Anne, Invercargill. New Zealand.

"My true being is expressing love, happiness and peace the entire day. It's like coming out of the darkness, into the light. It is like a fairy tale. I am a successful business woman standing with both feet in my life...very realistic. The difference is that now my work and my business are like play ... it is so beautiful. If people would know what it means to integrate spirituality and physicality, then life would be a dream. When we gain self confidence then love, peace and success is automatically following. This workshop showed me that we have powers but we just don't know how to tap into them. Denie shows us the way."

Maria, Vancouver Island, B.C. Canada.

"July 13th will always stand out as the most incredible experience I have ever had. There are no words to express the feeling. Thank you Denie and Shelley. When people ask about the group I have a hard time explaining because it was so special and I need to hold it close."

Frances, Mid-way, B.C. Canada.

"I'm just so thrilled with the freedom and confidence boost I am experiencing - I love seeing the effects of it on the people around me.... just an incredibly moving, profound and magical week!"

Jan, Vernon, B.C. Canada.

"During my life I have always been searching for what I believed to be the path and have tried many different disciplines. I have done what many would describe as dangerous hobbies but through Denie and his school I believe I have found MY path. Part of his school can be more terrifying than anything I have done before but also more satisfying, enlightening, and a beautiful cornucopia of esoteric teachings, and he presents them with an understanding and Mastery. Attending these schools has reaffirmed a belief that life isn't meant to be hard, it's supposed to be fun and it surely can be."

Dale, Fox Glacier. New Zealand.

"I feel as though, at some point between my late teens and early twenties I started to smother the sparks of light that were my life and joy, and without the sparks I got colder and colder until there was ice inside. The sparks are starting to glow now, and the ice is melting. I feel parts glowing with joy now that I had completely forgotten about and there are no words to describe this incredible feeling of coming alive again."

Michelle, Penticton, B.C. Canada.

"What a wild ride over here I'm having!! I realized it's important for me to make changes and so I began the day after I arrived home. Shelley I think of you sometimes as I'm skipping through the woods singing GOD I AM, I AM FREE, FREE TO BE TOTALLY ME! And Denie the meditations are excellent! My husband was so blown away with the changes in me after the IAVMS school he now wants to do it himself. Physically I feel more and more alive, I have reached a point now where I have had no pains whatsoever, and it definitely did not start like that. Very cool. I am hearing, seeing, and feeling everything in a very new way. I am !! I am said Sam! I am picking up messages every day in these ways this is incredibly helpful to me, and I love the answers and awareness I am receiving. Last night I felt like I stepped off a cliff, and instead of going into fear I thought, well I will either fly or there will be something solid to stand on, faith told me I would fly. I had an amazing day all day, I felt love whizzing out of every cell of my body. I felt like a human energy ball. I also put an ad in the paper for anyone with depression and anxiety to give me a call, I am talking to them about you. So many changes over here like black to white. I have the vision of learning much more of vibrational medicine from you. I am alive and vibrating."

Lorraine, Victoria, B.C. Canada.

"I now have an unlimited amount of energy, one week after my 2 week course. My food intake has been cut in half. I am positive and happy. The way Denie and Shelley planned and executed the courses is remarkable. I started to understand on the last day why they did it this way. I have high regards for both of them and this has to be taught to mankind. It is our God given right, as Denie would say, and I would not agree more. The sooner mankind wakes up the better for planet earth! All my love to Denie and Shelley, their work is remarkable."

Tjitske, Victoria, B.C. Canada.

"Best five day holiday I've ever had!"

Mike, Victoria, B.C., Canada

"Denie Hiestand, thank you, I have really enjoyed being in your company, you are a great crazy guy. I also want to say to you: thank you for the greatest gift you could give and have given me, which is your belief in me as a beautiful being. You have told me often and so forcefully that I have finally been able to make a start in believing it myself. Thank you."

Marian, Christchurch. New Zealand.

"WOW! Can't hardly believe it - my energy is increasing. I may have to abandon my morning coffee!"

Judy, Sidney, B.C. Canada.

"No more searching! I have found within me the compass needed to navigate through life with a knowing and awareness of my destination."

Elie, Victoria, B.C., Canada.

"An incredible way to wake up to all that you are! I now see things I had never yet seen, I hear things I had never listened for. I am going beyond every parameter and breaking free of all limitations I have put on myself. I have made a pact with myself that every time I see a heart I will tell myself how much I love "me." Since then the most incredible thing has happened... I see hearts everywhere! Amazing what happens when you raise your vibration! I am fine tuning the instrument that I am so that I may sing "My song" to the world. To Denie and Shelley - two incredible beings, two special friends, my heart thanks you, my soul thanks you. I share with you a quote from the I CHING Harmony Symbol, "Things that accord in tone vibrate together. Things that have affinity in their innermost natures seek one another." I encourage all of you to honor yourselves, to speak your truth and to follow your hearts."

Elaine, Victoria, B.C., Canada.

"The first module was outrageous. I loved the nature walk and seeing the lively energy. Since I have done this module I express myself better and love myself more. Denie and Shelley are fantastic people. I hope more kids my age take the course."

Janelle (age 12), Victoria, B.C., Canada.

INTERNATIONAL ACADEMY OF
VIBRATIONAL MEDICAL SCIENCE

PMB 654 15600 NE 8ᵗʰ St., B1
Bellevue, WA 98008

Ph. 425 785 3468
Fax 917 464 8128

E-mail: info@vibrationalmedicine.com
www.vibrationalmedicine.com

Registration of Interest Form

Dear Seeker,

It is with heartfelt joy that we invite you to apply to register your interest in the International Academy of Vibrational Medical Science.

Please fill out the form on next page and photocopy it and return it to **IAVMS Head Office** *at address above.*

Upon receipt of your registration we will send you confirmation of your registration, and all details of the dates, times and place that the school will be in session.
All students must start this program with the first module, Energy Awareness.
We look forward to sharing with you on your path of Expanded Awareness.

May you be blessed to find all that you seek.

INTERNATIONAL ACADEMY OF
VIBRATIONAL MEDICAL SCIENCE

REGISTRATION OF INTEREST DETAILS

NAME: _____

ADDRESS: _____

CITY: _____

STATE/PROV.: _____ ZIP/POSTAL: _____

COUNTRY: _____

PHONE: _____

E-MAIL: _____

FAX: _____

MALE/FEMALE: _____ DATE OF BIRTH: _____

SIGNED: _____

Journey to Truth

Denie Hiestand.
ISBN # 0-9684928-0-0, US$19.95
(First released as "Back to Life")

"This true story is not for the faint hearted. The author candidly discusses his struggle with the ongoing battle between ego and spirit. Compassionately, Denie's story shares answers in simple scientific terms about cosmic connections we as humans often find difficult to accept. Acts of unconditional love are woven into this inspirational message, pulling it all together with threads of self-improvement, inner awareness and esoteric teachings. If you're ready to remember who you are, JOURNEY TO TRUTH is a book you must read."

Personally recommended by
John Gray, Ph.D.
International best-selling Author of
Men are from Mars, Women are from Venus

Testimonials for "Journey to Truth"

"My highest personal recommendation!"

John Gray, PhD.
Author of Men are from Mars, Women are from Venus

"Journey to Truth is one man's inspiring and soul bearing story of his journey to truth and healing. More importantly, it is an introduction to the work of Denie Hiestand. As a medical doctor and student of Denie's International Academy of Vibrational Medical Science, the Christ force healing energy Denie teaches us to open our hearts to, is truly one of the most extraordinary, powerful, profound experiences of my entire life."

Dr. Linda C. Hole, MD. Spokane, WA. U.S.A.

"Somewhere in our hearts we each know that something more exists - some path that, once found, will explain, will exhilarate and will heal. Denie's journey takes you there. Journey to Truth irrevocably alters your life. It all becomes clear. A new kind of good is how you'll feel."

Linda, Durango, CO. U.S.A.

"Journey to Truth is an adventure story. It is also a story of spiritual transformation, an exciting account of innumerable precisely sequenced "coincidences" in the life of a charismatic New Zealand farmer, and the journey of a man who simply could not avoid his destiny as a remarkable healer and teacher."

Margaret, Sedona, AZ. U.S.A.

"In the words of Francis Bacon... "Some books are to be read in full and digested slowly." This is one whose full import does not hit one until long after they have closed the last pages. I needed to read this book twice with a month in between in order to realize that Journey to Truth is about being truly human in a way that everyone's being longs to be."

Cora, Kamloops, B.C. Canada.

"Yahoo! Finally a new book that will take people beyond the Celestine Prophesy - and it's true! Totally inspirational!"

Rio, Fall City, WA. U.S.A.

"The book every woman wants every man to read!"

Jan, Oliver, B.C. Canada.

"Journey to Truth does for men what Shirley McLaine's book Out on a Limb did for women. Finally we all have permission to feel."

Denise, Ashburton. New Zealand

"You could call me the world's biggest skeptic. However, Journey to Truth, got to me and changed my perceptions completely."

Radio John, Invercargill. New Zealand.

"Thankyou! Reading Journey to Truth affirmed for me many of my own experiences and helped me to see where I am heading more clearly."

Barbara, Kennebunk, ME.

"This year I gave myself the best Christmas present ever! I opened Journey to Truth at 8:00am on Christmas morning, thinking I would read a little of it before cooking Christmas dinner, and I couldn't put it down until I had finished it completely, at 7:00pm that night!"

Adell, Bellevue, WA. U.S.A.

"I haven't read a book for 20 years and I picked up Journey to Truth and couldn't put it down!"

Dennis, Salmon Arm, B.C. Canada.

"I've read a zillion books and it takes a lot to impress me. Journey to Truth is the first book I have read cover to cover, in one sitting, for eight years - it was that good!"

Jenni, Durango, CO. U.S.A.

"I am 84 years old and in all my years of living Journey to Truth is the book that has had the biggest impact on me. Every man should make this book compulsory reading. It contains all the messages we need for living. I have bought many copies of this book and given them to all my friends as Christmas presents to ensure that they read it."

Les, Salmon Arm, B.C. Canada.

"After sending away for your book (via USA) I have been anxiously waiting for 1 month.... I have just read up to page 20 in my lunch break - it has already brought me to tears (it is very powerful.... thank you I know that wait has been well worth it). Journey to Truth is just leaving me 'gob-smacked.' Absolutely incredible -it makes me laugh, cry, and I'm just awe-struck. I am clinging to each page·"

Ellen H., New Zealand.

"I just finished reading Denies book Journey to Truth. I am very thrilled as it describes exactly as I always felt our energy / spiritual system could work."

Peter M., Germany

"Just incredible. I hung on every page. I carried the book with me for a week, everywhere I went. Every moment I had, I opened it and read another page. The power I felt, such a deep truth. Thank you Denie for changing my life!"

Maria, Portland, ME

"Just last evening, I got home to find my copy of Journey to Truth had arrived. I read the first 5 chapters before I had to go to bed. I am giving your books to as many friends as I can think of. They are just eating them up!!!"

Gwen M., CA

"Your biography is one which really touches home to the various experiences that I also have journeyed. It is a book which made me excited because there you were, some stranger who identified my reality. Since that moment you spirit has been my inspiration.. May your spirits be blessed and may your journey be smiled upon by all of our Creator's spiritual essence."

Justin B., Whakatane, NZ

"Journey to Truth - a book that gives one hope for humanity".
Joey, Kelowna, B.C. Canada.

"I feel like I know you after reading Journey to Truth. I enjoyed the brisk way that I was able to read it. I also felt and cried at those incredible moments when you and your soul were communicating and you became aware of that fact. I also received a healing from the reading as I could feel the truth being told without embellishment. Your words carried an essence that entered me and gave me great hope of having a conscious connection with the incredible light of God."
Patricia Z., Seattle, WA

"Fabulous, fabulous, fabulous. I have read, as part of my work as a radio interviewer, every book anybody has written about spirituality and personal growth. Journey to Truth is the first book that tells it the way it is without embellishment, probably the most powerful read that I have ever had. Thank you Denie for telling it how it is. I unequivocally recommend this book to all my listeners. By the way, you are the most exciting, passionate guest I have ever had on my show."
Erskine Overnight, Phoenix, AZ

"I have just finished reading "Journey to Truth." I could not set it down! I have read through every part of it and have found it to be inspirational and exciting. I really related to Denie's feelings and experiences. His insight into spirituality and the world around us is extraordinary. I want to thank you two so much for showing the rest of us the light and the truth about who we really are.I am about to start on your book "Electrical Nutrition," and I am really excited to learn more about Vibrational medicine and electrical life. I am sure it will be a great experience for me. Take care, and thank Denie for his amazing work. I thoroughly enjoyed it."
Abe, Austin, TX

Testimonials for Electrical Nutrition.

"Dietetics describes in the old Greek world, 'the wholeness or the naturally correct behaviour of humans.' Electrical Nutrition, explains itself in the same way. A manual in life philosophy, it also teaches concepts in dietary intake. Nutrition, though decisive, is only a part of it. In reality, it is a question of consciousness, a slow process to which in this work, Denie and Shelley Hiestand provide a much needed, powerful, but logically presented stimulus. It is Electrical Nutrition for the body, mind and soul."

Peter Baumann, PhD. Basel. Switzerland.
Retired Head of Research, Novartis AG, Basel,. CH.

"In my nearly 20 years experience as an MD, Denie's work is truly remarkable. In my younger years, I studied honors physics with a Nobel laureate. Denie's work is likewise genius. Electrical Nutrition represents a paradigm shift in how we view the human body and dis-ease; and is a must for anyone interested in health and healing. I've had the honor and blessing to work clinically with Denie - with patients suffering from chronic pain, fibromyalgia, chronic fatigue, cancer, etc. Denie's clinical results are consistently astounding. . ."

Dr Linda C. Hole, MD. Spokane, WA, U.S.A.
Graduate Princeton and Duke Universities
Business Bureau Wholistic Doctor of the Year
American Academy of Pain Management
International Academy of Homeopathy
World QiGong Congress

"Reading Denie and Shelley's book Electrical Nutrition I am reminded of a favorite quote from Einstein: 'The problems that exist in the world today cannot be solved by the level of thinking that created them.' A different level of thinking produces ideas that make us uncomfortable, that push us out of our status quo stupor. Electrical Nutrition comes from a different level of thinking - it may make those of us trained in traditional western medicine very uncomfortable but I consider that a good thing. Like all of Denie and Shelley's work, this book is meant to shake us up, wake us up and get us moving down a different path - the path to an abundant, joy filled and absolutely radiant life.

Mary Pellicer, MD. Yakima WA. U.S.A.

"I highly recommend Electrical Nutrition to anyone interested in pursuing vibrant health and happiness."

John Gray, PhD.
Author of Men are from Mars, Women are from Venus.

"Congratulations! Great book!"

Dr. Kamnitzer
(personal friend of Dr. Gerber, author of Vibrational Medicine)

"We are vital energetic and super conscious beings leading a life of adventure and interest. We are presently 80+ years and growing younger by the year· We have both benefited from your great book Electrical Nutrition. Thank you!"

Ralph and Doreen C., Delta, BC, Canada.

"I am a Certified HOLISTIC Nutritional Consultant in California. I just started reading your book, am on page 25 and am totally compelled to email y'all. Again WOW! and thank you for doing this, I know I will be up all night finishing your "stuff." While reading only the first few pages my mind thinks of how many people I would like to see and read this book. This message needs to be heard ·I would like to preach your message to my many contacts in the nutrition world. I feel deeply in my heart that we can change the world, one baby step at a time. THANK YOU and Bless You for your book."

Diana R., Certified Nutrition Counselor, Newark, CA

"Thank you for the message to humanity which you are committed to serving up and for your example. The program you outline makes total sense. I pray I have the discipline to follow through and time to reprogram new healthy routines for myself."

Joyes B., San Francisco, CA

"I wish you all the best with this noble effort. You really have done your homework."

Julia Lacey, TV show Host, TX

"I would love Electrical Nutrition to be published in Spanish, my mother would benefit greatly from it·"

Marco M., Chatsworth, CA

"Thank you for your books, I had a good time reading them although I'm not sure I liked it very much especially when you said that it is OK to eat meat and the best meat was the human being· I was impressed with Denie and his life and the things that he went through to get to where he is now. What a story."

Samvado, India.

"I'm just about midway through reading your book about electrical nutrition (the info in it is common sense and no surprise to me!) and am very excited about "taking back" my health again. It's TIME TO HEAL!!!! I want to be "in" life again, w/out having to be in such horrendous pain and exhaustion."

Kelly S., Iowa

"I just sped-read your book last night.......I had chills and tears the entire time! WOW! I am so excited. Thank you for your work!"

Lynne, Chicago.

"Denie's insights, teachings, and supplements have boosted my health and consciousness to the next level. I feel better at 50 than ever before."

Bob, San Diego, CA.

"I've lost 20 pounds already, in one month, and everyone is commenting on how good I look. Everything is changing in my life and I feel on top of the world. Thank you."

Robert H., Long Hair Specialist to the Stars, Pasadena, CA.

"The content is phenomenal and controversial and makes real sense. It is information that must seep out into the hands of anyone even remotely interested in their health."

Jon, Durango, CO

"I have read Electrical Nutrition and was fascintated by it. There is a great deal of sense to it, and your background is helpful to establish its credibility, though it is indeed extreem to the common American perspective. If even a portion of your message takes hold it would be a good thing in this country. I wish you much success."

Laurie Harper, literary agent, St. Paul, MN

"My irritable bowel syndrome is gone, my husband's allergies are gone, we both feel so vibrant and alive, and our sex life has improved dramatically!"

Marilyn, Phoenix, AZ

"I was a strict vegan for 15 years and then I read your book. It really made me wake up. I have started to eat meat again, and I feel so good! Thank you!"

John, Nevada City, AZ

"Twenty years of abdominal pain and digestive discomfort disappeared within 3 days of following the advice in Electrical Nutrition. In the following 3 weeks, everything about my body, vitality, and my energy levels changed. I am 74 years of age and I never believed I could feel so good. I thought old age had set in and claimed my body, the logic in Electrical Nutrition told me that didn't have to happen and I am now living proof of that. I'm only buying one Christmas present this year and that is Electrical Nutrition for everyone I know. Thank you for giving me my body and my life back to me."

William W., Victoria, BC

"I've been into health and nutrition for the best part of 40 years, and this is the most logical, most common sense, all encompassing book I have ever read. I am part of a worldwide network of health professionals and therapists and we have put Electrical Nutrition on the top of our recommended reading list. This is the first health book that our organization has unequivocally recommended."

Paul, Subud, Victoria, BC, Canada.

"I've just read both your books and was blown away. This is incredible stuff."

Beth, LA

"The other morning while walking my dog, a neighbor drove up and commented on my weight loss. Now that really made my day! I must tell you both that I feel just fantastic. I've always been healthy, not fat, but healthy, and am blessed with good genes so I don't look my age. After reading 'Electrical Nutrition' I have changed my eating habits. I must tell you though that before reading this book, I had been on a 12 day cleansing fast, I won't do that again, especially after reading about the affects it can have, electrically. I can really tell a difference in the loss of fat when I'm not indulging in carbs and eating fruits, vegetables and protein. I find I don't have those cravings I use to have for carbs. It's simply amazing. I can even tell a difference in my hair and nails. I couldn't go into detail about how I lost the weight with my neighbor as she was on her way to dropping off her son and going to work, but this weekend I'll share the good news of your book, 'Electrical Nutrition' with her. By the way, I have changed my dog's diet (she certainly loves it). I will check with her vet about reducing her insulin intake."

Sheila, Minneapolis.

"I have been involved in the natural health industry for a long time and have had hundreds of books come my way - Electrical Nutrition makes the most sense of any book I have read and I recommend it to everyone."

Dr. Jackson Stockwell,
Health Professional and Radio Show Host, Utah.

"My food intake has been cut in half, I am positive and happy."

Tjitske, Holland.

"The cover itself sells the book - it was one of our best sellers when we displayed it on its own table in August."

Chapters Bookstore, Victoria, BC

"This book is going like hotcakes! The title and the cover are really catching people's attention. We have sold 60 copies in two weeks and the feedback about the book is great."

Open Secret Bookstore, San Rafael, CA

"I received 44 books at the International New Age Bookfair in Denver in June and Electrical Nutrition is the only one that jumped out at me and that I have read from cover to cover - I love it!"

Nancy Lee, Radio Show Host, Colorado.

"Every so often there's a new voice that entirely revitalizes and reinvents our perception of the body. Denie is such a person. We are grateful Denie has touched us."

Anna & Larry Halprin, California.

"I am a personal friend of Dr. Gerber - I noticed your book on the Internet - Congratulations! It is great to see more people writing about the Electrical Body."

David Kamnitzer

"I normally only ever read books associated with my business - Electrical Nutrition is the only book that has grabbed my attention for a long time. Every page has a gem on it."

Kelly, Yakima, WA

"I've just read Electrical Nutrition. Just amazing stuff - thank you!"

Mary, Vancouver

"At first I thought - just another health book - but once I started to read Electrical Nutrition I realized it has heaps of really good information in it that everyone should read."

Joe, Seattle

"Reading this book make sense and following its dietary guidelines, I am now able to wear clothing I have been unable to for the last two years - all this in three weeks! Everybody should read this book."

Ruth S., UT

"I couldn't sleep, got up loaded myself down with some heavy grains (ha, ha), and read on into your 'Electrical Nutrition' book, and feel inspired to write an infomercial at 12AM!! Oh, I already have a great start on the 60 second spot (a

couple more edits and this baby is gonna rock!!) the juice is flowin' and it ain't gonna turn off now. I am about to produce the greatest work of my life. I keep seeing bits and pieces of it from time to time (like a movie in my head.)"

Michael, Durango, CO

"I am a young student who, since I left home have kept gaining more and more weight. When I tried out the Electrical Nutrition suggestions I lost 30 pounds in 3 weeks."

Jeannie B., UT

"I've been a vegetarian since I was 15 yrs old, I couldn't believe when I started to suffer from the degenerative diseases that I thought I was immune to because of my "good diet." In my mid-50's I had already had two heart by-pass operations, blocked veins in my legs replaced, reproductive system operations and within ten years I was suffering once again from severe heart, breathing, circulatory and other health problems. I begged God to show me what I was doing wrong because I was still a staunch believer in my vegetarian ways but realized something was very wrong because I was dying from self-induced disease. In answer to my prayers my daughter told me to read a book called Electrical Nutrition. By the time I had finished the first chapter my emotions were welling up and I was shaking with the profound truth that the words were conveying to me. I stayed up all night reading and re-reading the book, battling with the concepts that were confronting what were my belief structures. Realizing I had begged God for answers to my serious health problems, and feeling an overwhelming deep truth I decided to try the dietary concepts contained within Electrical Nutrition. In the month that followed, everything about my body has changed. My weight has come down, my energy has gone up, I am off all my medication, and everything about my body that the medical profession said was unable to function again, is now coming back to life. My stomach is pain-free, my legs are pain-free and I am able to walk again, and every day I can move and feel and be in more and more joy. Electrical Nutrition has had the most unbelievable effect on myself and my family that I could ever have imagined. Thank you, thank you, thank you for having the courage to write this truth."

Nancy, Victoria, BC, Canada.

"I bought the book Electrical Nutrition and I finished reading it yesterday. I am still going in my mind over and over some of the principals, a lot of Great Information. I'm a massage therapist and very much interested in Vibrational medicine. Denie, you are going to need a body guard because of the things in this book are going to make some people very angry."

Douglas S., Phoenix, AZ

"Thank you so much for your wonderful presence at the Phoenix Whole Life Expo! I very much enjoyed meeting you and learning some more much needed details about my diet. I am enjoying the book greatly. You have such a fantastic sense of humor. All the best wishes on your journey and thank you for giving so much of yourself for the betterment of humanity!"

George, Phoenix, AZ

"After reading 'Electrical Nutrition' I must tell you that, I AM a Believer...Wow! Awesome words to digest, ingest, and just crave for more. Thank you."

Sheila

"A brilliant and timely book with unequivocal truths. This book should be on everyone's gift list this year. For years I suspected there was a fundamental truth missing from our current approach to medicine, nutrition and childbirth. Denie and Shelley have presented that truth in such a clear and definitive manner that you won't ever need to purchase another handbook for health."

Alex, WA

"Good book! I think this is one of those books where you read it and take what resonates with you from it. I did and lost 13 pounds just by doing the healthy eating recommendations. I also followed his recommendation of staying away from the middle isles at the supermarket because they are the ones with the food that has all the preservatives/toxins in the packaging. It worked for me. I feel a hell of a lot healthier and in tune to my body and what it needs. There is other good stuff in the book too. I would definitely tell someone to buy it."

IB, Saratoga, CA.

"Controversial must-read! The marketplace is flooded with books that discuss how to be healthy, how to improve spirituality and how to achieve enlightenment. Far too many of them ignore the impact of diet on these goals. We are a nation where 55% of the population is obese and where obesity is linked with severe health problems and early death. Despite this, medical and nutritional professionals are either ignorant of, or totally ignore, a plethora of research linking dietary practices to such problems. Too often, when they discuss diet, the present a narrow viewpoint, or glorify vegetarianism, which is not at all what people believe it to be. Denie Hiestand, the author of 'ELECTRICAL NUTRITION' argues that heavy reliance on grain (especially our beloved wheat), and use of preservatives (such deadly additives as MSG and Aspartame) are major causes for destroying the health of our bodies and dimming our spiritual lights. He also discusses vegetarianism, immunizations, the birthing process and other cultural practices that keep us from achieving our goals regarding health and enlightenment. Finally, as a psychologist, I have noticed how much better people function when they take a close look at their dietary practices. I have also been amazed at the results when Denie and I work with people with respect to all aspects of their electrical functioning. In brief, if you seek to guide yourself to better emotional and physical health, this book must be read!"

Dr. Stephen Vizzard, Bellevue, WA.

"This book makes you go dah! It spells everthing out. When I first started to make my way through this book, I was thinking this guy is a little off his rocker in the statements he makes until I started to think about it. It took a couple of days but after I thought about what he had said, it kinda made me think about the perspective I have on the world and realized where it came from. I see things how I was told to think. Not the way they truly are. This book rocks!"

Aaron, Spokane, WA

"Challenged my beliefs about diet & medicine. An eye opener! The author is knowledgeable and gets right to the point. Many important questions are raised. I am shocked when I realize the effect on my body of processed 'food-shaped products', I am thankful to this author for the challenging my beliefs. Some of the language seems overly critical and extreme, but reasonable solutions are provided, and when I suspended my reactions I could let the good stuff sink in. Share your copy with your MD and see what s/he does with it."

AB, Victoria, BC

BOOK & AUDIO ORDERS

Electrical Nutrition; ISBN # 0-968428-1-9
By Denie & Shelley Hiestand   **US $14.95**

Electrical Nutrition Audio; ISBN # 0-968428-4-3
By Denie & Shelley Hiestand   **US $29.95**

Journey to Truth; ISBN # 0-9684928-0-0
By Denie Hiestand   **US $19.95**

All orders plus shipping, handling and taxes.

Individual Credit Card Orders please phone

1 800 207 2239

or **403 314 2351**

if calling outside US or Canada.

New Zealand Book Orders:
Call Nationwide Books 0 800 990 123 or 03 366 9559

All other orders please contact the Publisher

Mailing Address Only

ShellDen Publishing
PMB 654 15600 NE 8th St., B1
Bellevue, WA 98008

Ph. 425 785 3468
Fax 917 464 8128

E-mail: info@vibrationalmedicine.com
www.vibrationalmedicine.com

Where to and How: page

How to contact us:

Mailing Address Only

ShellDen Publishing
PMB 654 15600 NE 8th St., B1
Bellevue, WA 98008

Ph. 425 785 3468
Fax 917 464 8128

E-mail: info@vibrationalmedicine.com
www.vibrationalmedicine.com